Patient-Centered Clinical Care for African Americans

Gregory L. Hall

Patient-Centered Clinical Care for African Americans

A Concise, Evidence-Based Guide to Important Differences and Better Outcomes

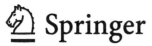 Springer

Gregory L. Hall, MD
Partnerships for Urban Health
Cleveland State University
Cleveland, OH
USA

ISBN 978-3-030-26417-8   ISBN 978-3-030-26418-5   (eBook)
https://doi.org/10.1007/978-3-030-26418-5

This Springer imprint is published by the registered company Springer Nature Switzerland AG
The registered company address is: Gewerbestrasse 11, 6330 Cham, Switzerland

*This book is dedicated to my wife, Melanie,
and our sons, Alex, Nick, and Greg Jr., for all
of their sacrifice and unwavering support.*

Preface

In the fall of 2002, I was appointed to the Ohio Commission on Minority Health. My name had been submitted to Ohio Governor Bob Taft by Cleveland's Mayor Jane Campbell because they needed a medical professional from the Cleveland area to better balance the representation to the state-wide board. As a Cleveland Clinic-trained internal medicine and primary care provider in an urban practice that was over 90% African American, I could provide in-the-trenches perspectives. Upon joining, I was embarrassed to admit how little I knew about health disparities and how they impacted minorities, but I attended the meetings regularly ... and quietly.

The commission was largely a funding organization and specialized in advancing smaller grants for unique approaches to shrinking health disparities. We also advocated for policies that impact health in the larger scheme. The commission is composed of the directors of key statewide departments including the Departments of Health, Job and Family Services, Education, Medicaid, Developmental Disabilities, and Mental Health and Addiction, in addition to four elected officials and eight governor appointees, of which I was one.

Bringing a "high-end" group like this together was initially intimidating but before long we began to fill our roles appropriately. As a physician, I initially believed that health disparities were almost completely driven by poverty and/or the lack of access to medical services. I also falsely believed that "minorities" had poor health outcomes and the "majority" populations had better health outcomes.

Because of my work with the commission, I soon joined the Medical Care Advisory Committee for Ohio Medicaid. In this capacity, I saw not only the financial burden that poor health outcomes put on a strained state budget but also the disconnect between providers of Medicaid recipients and state agency representatives with good intentions.

My exposure to the breadth of urban healthcare delivery was rounded by my experience as medical director of multiple urban extended care facilities including two with large psychiatric populations, continued inpatient care with patients at an inner city hospital (St. Vincent Charity Medical Center), and some time as medical director of home health and hospice agencies.

As the years passed, I was elected vice-chair and then chairman of the Ohio Commission on Minority Health. A part of my duties was to prepare an educational chairman's report to be presented at each meeting. As I became familiarized with research articles involving quality outcomes, I was struck by the significant health disparities *between* minority groups and that the specific health issues were not addressed by the same solutions. Problems in the Asian American or Hispanic/ Latino communities consisted of issues regarding immigration, communication, language, and access. African American disparities were pervasive across a range of categories: the worst cardiovascular issues, worst cancer outcomes, longest length of hospital stay, lowest referrals for accelerated care, and so on. Put simply, the health-related problems for African Americans were too serious, too unique, and too severe to simply be "bunched" with other racial/ethnic groups.

My second revelation was that physicians, clinicians, and other providers were indirectly contributing to some of these disparities. This perspective was first brought to my attention by the Commission Executive Director Cheryl Boyce, who had noted these differences from both a professional and a personal perspective. I remember initially shrugging off her viewpoint as isolated because variability in care delivery can occur, but when I reviewed the wide-ranging research, the pervasive clinician-driven differences in the care of African Americans were undeniable.

I decided to highlight some of these care differences on my practice website, drgreghall.com, in order to educate the African American community to be better stewards of their medical care. As I composed these short articles with hyperlinks to verified research in PubMed, I was progressively finding more nuances in clinical care.

I realized that my aim to educate about the differences in the clinical care of African Americans was directed to the wrong audience, and I needed to move "upstream" and bring these differences to the notice of medical providers. That realization soon led to the process of compiling a collection of best practices for African American clinical care, one that is long overdue and deserving of the medical community's singular attention.

Cleveland, OH, USA   Gregory L. Hall, MD
June 18, 2019

Acknowledgments

This book was definitely a group effort and the culmination of a number of partnerships and affiliations across my career. I started the book by interviewing a number of highly successful physicians who had predominant African American patient populations. As a provider for African Americans, I knew that my approach to this patient population was different, but I needed to know if there was a distinct pattern. I particularly appreciate the input of Ronald Adams, MD; Lloyd Cook, MD; Giesele Greene, MD; Carl Jackson, MD; Toye Williams, MD; and Harold James, MD, for their assistance early on. I also need to thank my brother, Bill Hall, for introducing me to his physician colleagues for interviews in the Maryland region including Elmer Carreno, MD; Geoff Mount-Varner, MD; and Don Shell, MD. Another important interview was with my good friend since our Cleveland Clinic residency days, Mark Spears, MD, in Florida.

Many thanks to my colleagues and the staff at St. Vincent Charity Medical Center including Chief Medical Officer Joseph Sopko, MD, one of the earliest reviewers; Department of Medicine Chairman Keyvan Ravakha, MD; and supportive colleagues, Mukul Pandit, MD; Donald Eghobamien, MD; Sam Ballesteros, MD; Alan Rosenfield, MD; Mona Reed, MD; Jill Barry, MD; James Boyle, MD; John Marshall, MD; Emmanuel Elueze, MD; Oluwaseun Opelami, MD; and Lonnie Marsh, MD.

The residency program at St. Vincent Charity Medical Center produces topnotch physicians who also contributed to this book. Randol Kennedy, MD, and Anita Mason-Kennedy, MD, reviewed and added to the entire book with particular contributions to the chapters on cardiology, hematology, and rheumatology. I also appreciate and thank graduate Medical Education Manager Nicole Allen-Banks. Other residents proofreading include Nana Yaa, MD, and Adeyinka Owoyele, MD.

My cousin, Kim Simpson, MD, was my first reviewer and got this book off to a great start particularly contributing to the first three chapters. Good friend Joan Reeder, MD, also reviewed the book early on.

I was honored to have the chapters on cardiovascular and renal disease reviewed with significant input by Jackson T. Wright Jr., MD, PhD. Sherrie Dixon-Williams, MD, reviewed and contributed to the pulmonary chapter.

I appreciate the ongoing support of Janet Baker, DNP, dean of Ursuline College School of Nursing, for her support in reviewing the book. The chapter on stories and patient counseling was reviewed by William Tarter Sr., and I appreciate his ongoing guidance and counsel.

I would also like to express my gratitude to Cheryl and Russel Boyce; Nick and Yvette Petty; Thomas Ferkovic; Georgia State Senator Emanuel Jones; Georgia State Rep. Al Williams; Donald Wesson, MD, MBA; John McCarthy; Charles Modlin, MD; Angela Cornelius Dawson; Cora Munoz, PhD, RN; Danny Williams; Deborah Enty; Mary E. Weems, PhD; Michael Oatman; Reggie Blue, PhD; Paul Lecat, MD; David Whitaker, JD; Tim Goler, PhD; Robert Ankrum; Ronald Duncan; Robert Dennison; Earl King; Terry Ford; Alana Smith; and a host of other physicians, nurses, and professionals with whom I work in various capacities.

My office practice would not be able to stay afloat without my office manager, Robin Smith, holding everything together. Medical Assistant Jasmine Williams always has a happy and caring smile for both my patients and I. My long-term administrative assistant, Katrina Hurt, also deserves credit for her support over the years. I am also grateful to my patients who have supported my work and encouraged me. My patients are the best in the world, and I treasure their support and commitment.

My position as co-director of the Northeast Ohio Medical University-Cleveland State University Partnership for Urban Health has allowed me to work with an outstanding array of people. My predecessor in this position is a modern medicine legend and is dedicated to excellence and inclusion in all he does, Edgar Jackson Jr., MD. Ronnie Dunn, PhD, is an outstanding leader in diversity and inclusion and was very instrumental in getting this book published. Celeste Ribbons is an outstanding operations manager, organizer, and counselor. Lena Grafton is an excellent teacher, researcher, and outreach officer. Antoinette Speed does a great job keeping us organized and successful in our projects. Peggy Irwin is an outstanding grant writer, teacher, and manager. Dr. Julian Earls has been a constant inspiration to me and is a champion among educators. School of Health Sciences Director Beth Domholdt is the perfect collaborator due to her insight, experience, and compassion. Dean Meredith Bond of the College of Sciences and Health Professions has also been very supportive of our work and has great intuition and knowledge. My sincere thanks also go to the provost of Cleveland State University, Jianping Zhu, PhD.

I am an active faculty member at the Northeast Ohio Medical University College of Medicine and appreciate the support provided by my department chairs, Joseph Zarconi, MD, and William Chilian, PhD. I also thank the leadership of the College of Medicine Dean Elisabeth Young, MD, and Vice Dean Eugene Mowad, MD. I also recognize the talents of my co-director, Sonja Harris-Haywood, MD.

Having been on the Cuyahoga County Board of Health for almost 10 years, I have had the opportunity to see how a world-class public health entity can work. Its commissioner, Terrence Allan, was instrumental in my initial appointment and has always been supportive, inclusive, and incredibly productive. We have a great team at CCBH lead by our board president, Debbie Moss-Batt, and my fellow board members, Jim Gatt, Doug Wang, and Sherrie Williams, MD.

Working with the Saber Healthcare Group and its leaders, George Repchick and Bill Weisberg, has been a highlight of my career, and I sincerely appreciate their support and encouragement throughout our many years together. I also appreciate Gia Weisberg and Lynda Repchick for their support as well as Grant and Lisa Weimer.

My high school classmates, Kevin Goldsmith, JD; Martin Davidson, PhD; and Henry Butler from University School also helped greatly through advice and counsel. My Williams College classmates, Ray Headen, JD, Deborah Marcano, and Peter Graffagnino, also contributed support through networking and advice.

Thanks to Richard Lansing for his support throughout the publishing process and for immediately seeing the potential of this book.

And finally, thanks to the Hall family, my mother and father (Louise and Albert Hall) who supported me unconditionally and my brothers and sister, Tyrone, Wanda, Bill, and Barry, who always made sure I was loved and nurtured. With marriage comes my extended family that has also been supportive including my sisters-in-law, Robin, Stacie, and Lorraine, and my brother-in-law, Sherman, who have always provided expert counsel and advice. My wife Melanie's side of the family has also been supportive and accepting, and I will always treasure my mother- and father-in-law, Mamie and Jesse Coats, as well as my brother-in-law, Michael, and sister-in-law, Valeri. I love and thank all of our nieces and nephews and the rest of the Hall and Coats families. Other supportive family members include Martin Kelly; Jeff Johnson, JD; Duane Morton; Geovette (GiGi) Houston; Tony Whitaker; Cynthia Simpson; Cheryl Staples; Lynette Bennet; Judith Dunn; and our great friends, Paul and Valencia Stephens.

It truly took a village to get this book written and published.

Contents

Why Is Patient-Centered Culturally Competent Care Important?

1

Despite countless social and societal norms, we are all different. Having a book that advances generalizations based on race or ethnicity can be a risky and potentially inflammatory endeavor. Whenever you generalize about people, there are going to be glaring exceptions that can be embarrassing, hurtful to the patient, and, above all, counter-productive. I remember asking an 80-year-old new patient what her mother died from. And seeing the look on her face, that initially suggested I knew something that she did not. And her reply was "my 97-year-old mother was fine when I left her this morning."

On the positive side, some generalizations can consistently be assumed. The *patient-centered* movement has placed respect and consideration of the patient as a central tenet, and it would be hard to find those who would disagree with this approach.

It is important to note that I am fully aware of the "danger" of classifying a race/ethnic group as homogenous. Chinedu Ejike discussed these potential inaccuracies in his article about chronic obstructive pulmonary disease (COPD) in America's "Black" population:

> Currently, Blacks in America are a rapidly growing subset of the U.S. population and the growing black immigrant population has recently fueled this growth. COPD prevalence and morbidity vary widely among African Americans (U.S. born blacks) versus black immigrants (foreign-born blacks), but most studies have treated blacks in America as a homogeneous "African-American" population. This assumption ignores the disparities in socioeconomic status, tobacco or biomass smoke exposure, social behaviors, access to healthcare, health insurance coverage and disease management present among the subgroups of blacks in America. The use of "African American" to describe all U.S. blacks in the majority of observational and interventional studies should be avoided and better

© Springer Nature Switzerland AG 2020

G. L. Hall, *Patient-Centered Clinical Care for African Americans*,

https://doi.org/10.1007/978-3-030-26418-5_1

stratification performed in studies moving forward to allow for the design of effective preventive and therapeutic interventions. [1]

Dr. Ejike is completely correct, and his view represents the perspective of many providers and researchers. A more nuanced approach would definitely be more appropriate. This book, however, cites "evidence-based" research where "differences" based on race/ethnicity existed however it was defined. When population differences did not achieve statistical significance, it was likely because of the heterogenicity inherent in almost any racial/ethnic group in the United States. In order for differences to exist, a statistical difference had to exist, and with African American health differences, many of these differences are unequivocal.

This book is thin because in the world of medicine, humans are far more alike than different. Many of the important differences in the care of African Americans involve giving more attention to certain details of their care. Screen more vigilantly for cancer, spend more time on smoking cessation, think about lupus, sarcoidosis, and other rare disorders when you are frustrated by an odd patient presentation. This approach is no different than "thinking of Lyme disease" when a patient presents with complaints after camping in New England. Lyme disease can be transmitted in numerous places across the United States, but providers are trained to particularly look for oddball diseases in these cases because the likelihood is supposed to be higher.

Some of the important differences we see in African Americans are based on minor genetic differences like sickle cell anemia and others. Other differences are based on diet, environmental exposures, poverty, lifestyle choices, and more. These differences are not to be applied blindly to every patient you see, but instead are to be "considered." By simply considering these important differences, improved clinical care outcomes across a population will ensue.

The Institute of Medicine's *Unequal Treatment: Confronting Racial and Ethnic Disparities in Health Care* section on cross-cultural communication describes the benefit:

> Sociocultural differences between patient and provider influence communication and clinical decision-making. Evidence suggests that provider-patient communication is directly linked to patient satisfaction, adherence, and subsequently, health outcomes. Thus, when sociocultural differences between patient and provider aren't appreciated, explored, understood, or communicated in the medical encounter, the result is patient dissatisfaction, poor adherence, poorer health outcomes, and racial/ethnic disparities in care. And it is not only the patient's culture that matters; the provider "culture" is equally important. Historical

factors for patient mistrust, provider bias, and its impact on physician decision-making have also been documented. Failure to take sociocultural factors into account may lead to stereotyping, and in the worst cases, biased or discriminatory treatment of patients based on race, culture, language proficiency, or social status. [2]

After reviewing countless research articles and interviewing numerous physicians, there are clear clinical differences between racial and ethnic communities that allow some generalizations that can be impactful in the clinical setting. Some of these differences are based on poverty, education, or urban environment, while others are more lifestyle-related and based on local community norms (smoking, diet, or lack of exercise). Advances in genetics and epigenetics are also highlighting differences that can impact the course or severity of a number of diseases.

Alexis Vick and Heather Burris at Harvard University described the potential impact of social and environmental exposures and the epigenetic pathophysiologic consequences:

Epigenetic mechanisms, particularly DNA methylation, can be altered in response to exposures such as air pollution, psychosocial stress, and smoking. Each of these exposures has been linked to the above health states (cardiovascular disease, cancer, and preterm birth) with striking racial disparities in exposure levels. DNA methylation patterns have also been shown to be associated with each of these health outcomes.... Whether DNA methylation mediates exposure-disease relationships and can help explain racial disparities in health is not known. However, because many environmental and adverse social exposures disproportionately affect minorities, understanding the role that epigenetics plays in the human response to these exposures that often result in disease, is critical to reducing disparities in morbidity and mortality. [3]

In an article by Vivian Chou at Harvard University "How Science and Genetics are Reshaping the Race Debate of the 21st Century," she explains that racial differences based on genetic variation are practically nonexistent. It is important to note that genetic differences across all races are remarkably small; she writes that "in the biological and social sciences, the consensus is clear: race is a social construct, not a biological attribute" [4]. In fact, as a species humans are "99.9% identical in their genetic makeup" [5].

Despite the wide-spread genetic similarity described, there are undeniable and statistically significant differences in health outcomes for African Americans. As the root cause of these differences becomes clearer, it is important for providers to stay abreast of the latest trends and distinctions.

1.1   Pay for Performance

Any time spent trying to find ways to better care for patients is advantageous, and now, thanks to provider "pay-for-performance" outcome measurements, more competently treating individual patients will directly drive our income potential [6–8].

If considered selfishly, poor patient outcomes will drag down our "accountability scores," influence our reimbursement and preferred status with insurances, and jeopardize our ability to make a living. More globally, by ignoring potential differences that impact clinical outcomes, we are negatively affecting health disparities and decreasing the quality of the care we provide.

The Agency for Healthcare Research and Quality (AHRQ) looked at hospitalizations by race/ethnicity and then stratified the outcome by income and found that *in all income groups*, the rates of potentially avoidable hospitalizations were higher for African Americans than European Americans. In fact, European Americans in the lowest income groups had lower rates of avoidable hospitalizations than the richest African Americans [9] (Fig. 1.1).

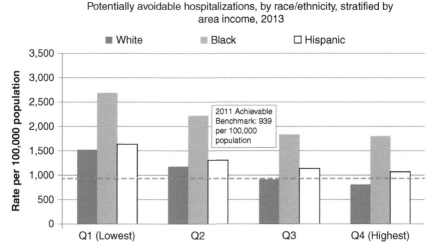

Potentially avoidable hospitalizations, by race/ethnicity, stratified by area income, 2013

Key: Q = quartile. based on the median income of a patient's ZIP Code of residence
Source: Agency for Healthcare Research and Quality (AHRQ), Healthcare Cost and Utilization Project, State Inpatient Databases, 2013 quality and disparities analysis file, and AHRQ Quality Indicators, modified version 4.4
Note: Rates are adjusted by age and gender using the total U.S. resident population for 2010 as the standard population

Fig. 1.1 Potentially avoidable hospitalizations. Chartbook on Health Care for Blacks: National Healthcare Quality and Disparities Report. https://www.ahrq.gov/research/findings/nhqrdr/chartbooks/blackhealth/acknow.html

Most providers acknowledge the existence of health disparities and unequal care when looking outward at the world, the United States, or their immediate community. The problem occurs when individual physicians have to come to terms with their personal contribution to health disparities [10]. In a sense, many believe unequal care occurs, but *just not when they are around*. To accept that you might be contributing to unequal care is a big step and can be a professional revelation.

Many minority clinicians falsely believe that because they are minorities, they cannot contribute to health disparities. They believe that through a birthright, they automatically treat everyone appropriately. Not true. A lack of knowledge of clinical differences in patient populations you treat results in inferior care. Anyone of any race or ethnicity can have a lack of knowledge. Learning about the cultural perspective of a patient and the research-verified clinical care differences allows us to better connect, adapt our interventions appropriately, and positively impact clinical outcomes.

The recent expansion of research based on detailed genetic mapping has allowed for significant advances in our understanding of why some medications or clinical approaches work in some patients and not in others. Considerations like salt sensitivity, which impacts less than 50% of the overall American population, affect over 70% of African Americans [11, 12]. These differences offer significantly alternative approaches to population health. Genetic and epigenetic differences that affect the level of kidney disease, severity of cancer, level of cholesterol, risk for stroke or obesity, and much more have all been identified and shown to be significantly different in African Americans.

Knowing about and implementing clinical care that is carefully tailored to your patient population will require additional time and effort, but that energy will be saved in the more efficient control of hypertension, reduction of obesity, anticipation and prevention of cancers, and countless other approaches that will undeniably improve your clinical care.

1.2 Patient-Centered Care

In 1988, the Picker Institute coined the term "patient-centered care" as a way to move medical care back to its roots where physicians provided compassionate and personalized care to a patient before applying an array of diagnostic technologies that moved the physician away from direct patient involvement [13]. Patient-centered care, as reported by the Institute of Medicine, is one of the six key elements of high-quality care listed in their landmark "Crossing the Quality Chasm" report of 2002 [14]. This medical expert-driven report stresses that healthcare should be:

1. *Safe*—avoiding injuries to patients from the care that is intended to help them
2. *Effective*—providing services based on scientific knowledge to all who could benefit and refraining from providing services to those not likely to benefit (avoiding underuse and overuse)
3. *Patient-centered*—providing care that is respectful of and responsive to individual patient preferences, needs, and values and ensuring that patient values guide all clinical decisions
4. *Timely*—reducing waits and sometimes harmful delays for both those who receive and those who give care
5. *Efficient*—avoiding waste, in particular waste of resources
6. *Equitable*—providing care that does not vary in quality because of personal characteristics such as gender, ethnicity, geographic location, and socioeconomic status

As healthcare continues to be transformed, placing the patient back into the focus of care has been a central tenet.

With African Americans representing 13% of the total US population and over 45 million people [15], learning about the culturally driven healthcare issues that this population faces is time well spent. African Americans in some urban areas make up greater than 50% of patients at a given hospital. To not spend any time learning about their cultural foundations as a people, and their racial or ethnic clinical care idiosyncrasies, is a recipe for poor patient outcomes. Having patient-centered care as a quality measure has both simplified and complicated the dilemma that cultural competence presented.

In 1985 the Health and Human Resources Secretary under President Ronald Reagan, Margaret Heckler, formed the Secretary's Task Force on Black and Minority Health [16]. This "Heckler Report" would for the first time legitimize the notion that African Americans were suffering from persistent health disparities that accounted for excess morbidity and mortality. This report inspired the formation of the US Office on Minority Health and state-based Commissions on Minority Health.

In 1998 Jeffrey T. Berger wrote "Culture and Ethnicity in Clinical Care" for the Journal of the American Medical Association and stressed the importance of "physician recognition of the cultural context of patients' illnesses (that) can be essential to a successful therapeutic relationship" [17]. Soon after, the term cultural competence [18] began to reflect a practitioner's "ability to interact effectively with people of different cultures." It essentially meant being respectful and responsive to the health beliefs and practices—and cultural and linguistic needs—of diverse population groups. Developing cultural competence was seen as an evolving, dynamic process that occurred along a continuum.

Scholars and practitioners questioned the futility of placing any particular patient in a cultural category with any degree of precision [19]. Moreover, anthropologists and sociologists wondered if a person from one culture could truly become "competent" in another culture and maintain it over time. Most agreed that achieving "cultural competence" in multiple cultures was likely futile due to the pure volume of information to master.

Within a couple of years, the concept and benefits of patient-centered care began to take hold. Patient-centered care results in a better perception of the quality of care, improved health status (less discomfort, less concern, and better mental health), and increased efficiency of care (reduced diagnostic tests and referrals) as reported in a study by Stewart et al. [19]. They found that patients had the impression of improved health based on "being a full participant in the discussions during the encounter" which led to better trust in their providers.

The Picker Institute [13] advanced principles that have widely been accepted as cornerstones of patient-centered care:

1. Respect for patients' values, preferences, and expressed needs
2. Coordination and integration of care
3. Information, communication, and education
4. Physical comfort
5. Emotional support and alleviation of fear and anxiety
6. Involvement of family and friends
7. Continuity and transition
8. Access to care

African Americans have been the recipients of population-centered care. Well-meaning practitioners from across the country have insisted that the American experience culturally provided enough customization for African Americans. One burning question remained. Why were African American clinical outcomes so poor with such significant disparities?

If the cultural experience were the same (or even similar) across Americans, providing cultural care in a standardized fashion would make sense. But from a healthcare standpoint, the cultural differences between African Americans and European Americans are stark. Historically African Americans have not had equal access. Instead, inferior care was accepted, and there was experimentation, exclusions from hospitals, and abuse of African American bodies both living and dead. These substantive historical differences greatly impact African American's perspective of the medical field in general, and of providers in particular.

The disparate treatment of the African American poor and disenfranchised throughout the history of slavery, poverty, and civil rights transgressions is unfortunate, yet undeniable, facts in American history. To ignore that cultural history and the stories of those not-too-distant events and pretend that modern-day African Americans are minimally influenced by, those events is wishful thinking at best.

The study and published article "Race and Trust in the Health Care System" looked specifically at the perspectives African Americans had regarding medical research, healthcare, and physician providers, when compared to European Americans [20]. African Americans were less likely to trust their physicians, and more likely to be concerned about personal privacy and harmful experimentation. Thus, there are patterns of distrust of our healthcare system among African Americans that impact their acceptance of our advice, comfort with our use of their personal information, and a suspicion of our motives to help. This is in stark contrast to European Americans who, by and large, do not come to the table with these concerns [21]. Generally, European Americans have good impressions of the medical care delivered by physicians and nurses, and there is minimal, if any, history of experimentation, collusion, or neglect for this population in America. The two resulting perspectives, one of implicit trust and confidence and the other with mistrust and suspicions of motives, provide a dramatically contrasting patient base that will require differing approaches to establishing a successful patient-physician relationship.

To accept the events of America's medical and clinical past is at times painful because we have been trained to believe that our medical profession is the best in the world, and it is. But being the best does not make it flawless. Being the best does not erase the countless indecencies suffered by African Americans. But acknowledging the past, and adjusting our care based on that past medical history, is a sound and beneficial approach to the care of a historically abused people.

The ensuing chapters will briefly review an approach to the patient-centered care of African Americans that "considers" their cultural and racial past, as well as recent data suggesting best practices in clinical care. These best practices are merely the customization of clinical decisions to the African American race. As researchers find progressively more differences in the genetics and epigenetics of heart disease, specific cancers, approaches to pharmacological therapy, and others that are different in African Americans from European Americans, thought leaders are now proclaiming (with decreasing health disparities in mind) that there are a number of clear and impactful differences in clinical care that merit all clinicians' notice.

From the genetic mutational profiles of prostate and breast cancers that make them more aggressive to the genomic risk prediction models for common diseases that allow for early detection and more efficient treatment, genetic scientists across the world are uncovering a wealth of clinical nuances that can greatly impact quality care and outcomes in African Americans.

Why Is Patient-Centered Culturally Competent Care Important?
- It positively impacts patient encounters.
- It positively impacts your quality measures.
- It positively impacts insurance reimbursement.
- It positively improves your patient's perception of the quality of their care and improves compliance with orders and medications.

References

1. Ejike CO, Cransfield MT, Hansel NN, et al. Chronic obstructive pulmonary disease in America's black population. Am J Respir Crit Care Med. 2019;200(4):423–30. https://doi.org/10.1164/rccm.201810-1909PP.
2. Smedley BD, Stith AY, Nelson AR, editors. Unequal treatment: confronting racial and ethnic disparities in health care. Washington: The National Academies Press; 2003. p. 200–1.
3. Vick AD, Burris HH. Epigenetics and health disparities. Curr Epidemiol Rep. 2017;4(1):31–7.
4. Chou V. How science and genetics are reshaping the race debate of the 21st century. Science in the news. Harvard University. The Graduate School of Arts and Sciences. http://sitn.hms.harvard.edu/flash/2017/science-genetics-reshaping-race-debate-21st-century/. Accessed 5 May 2019.
5. Genetics vs. genomics fact sheet. National Human Genome Research Institute. https://www.genome.gov/about-genomics/fact-sheets/Genetics-vs-Genomics. Accessed 5 May 2019.
6. Rosenthal MB, Frank RG, Li Z, Epstein AM. Early experience with pay-for-performance: from concept to practice. JAMA. 2005;294:1788–93.
7. Rosenthal MB. Beyond pay for performance--emerging models of provider-payment reform. New Engl J Med. 2008;359:1197–200.
8. Bond AM, Volpp KG, Emanual EJ, et al. Real-time feedback in pay-for-performance: Does more information lead to improvement? J Gen Inter Med. 2019;34(9):1737–43. https://doi.org/10.1007/s11606-019-05004-8.
9. 2015 national healthcare quality and disparities report chartbook on health care for blacks. Rockville: Agency for Healthcare Research and Quality; 2016. AHRQ Pub. No 16-0015-1-EF.
10. Kendrick J, Nuccio E, Leiferman JA, Sauaia A. Primary care providers' perceptions of racial/ethnic and socioeconomic disparities in hypertension control. Am J Hypertens. 2015;28(9):1091–7.

11. Luft FC, Grim CE, Higgins JT Jr, Weinberger MH. Differences in response to sodium administration in normotensive white and black subjects. J Lab Clin Med. 1977;90(3):555–62.
12. Madhavan S, Alderman MH. Ethnicity and the relationship of sodium intake to blood pressure. J Hypertens. 1994;12(1):97–103.
13. Picker Institute. Retrieved from http://www.ipfcc.org/resources/picker-institute.html. Accessed 6 May 2019.
14. Institute of Medicine (US) Committee on Quality Care in America. Crossing the quality chasm: a new health system for the 21st century. Washington: National Academies Press (US); 2001.
15. United States Census Bureau. Retrieved from https://www.census.gov/quickfacts/fact/table/US. Accessed 6 May 2019.
16. "The heckler report: a force for ending health disparities in America." Retrieved from https://minorityhealth.hhs.gov/heckler30/. Accessed 6 May 2019.
17. Berger J. Culture and ethnicity in clinical care. Arch Intern Med. 1998;158(19):2085–90.
18. Cultural competence. https://www.samhsa.gov/capt/applying-strategic-prevention/cultural-competence. Accessed 6 May 2019.
19. Stewart M, Brown J, Donner A, et al. The impact of patient-centered care on outcomes. J Fam Pract. 2000;49(9):796–804.
20. Boulware L, Cooper L, Ratner L, LaVeist T, Powe N. Race and trust in the health care system. Public Health Rep. 2003;118:358.
21. Halbert C, Armstrong K, Gandy O, Shaker B. Racial differences in trust in health care providers. Arch Intern Med. 2006;166(8):896–901.

Establishing Trust

2

Multiple studies over an extended period of time confirm what most clinicians already knew, African Americans are generally not as trusting of medical providers as other racial groups [1, 2]. What many of us did not know was why. As providers, we spent many years training to help others. Medicine is a service profession. Why would anyone suspect our intentions, question our motives, or assign us collectively as untrustworthy? The answer lies in the historical experience African Americans had with America's doctors, hospitals, and researchers.

Before delving into ways to build trust, it is imperative to have a perspective as to why the trust that most of the majority population has for the field of medicine is lost to many African Americans. And why, despite the fact that many of these historical atrocities occurred to people other than today's patients, the stories and suspicions are passed from one generation to the next.

2.1 The Tuskegee Syphilis Study

The Tuskegee Syphilis Study was originally formed to record the natural history of syphilis with the hope of justifying the funding of public treatment programs for African Americans. The study, which began in 1932, included 600 African American men, 399 with syphilis and 201 without the disease [3, 4]. While the study was originally slated to last 6 months, it was extended for over 40 years. Penicillin became widely available in 1942 as an accepted curative treatment for syphilis, but the researchers wanted to gain more information about untreated syphilis so the participants were neither informed nor treated. Central to the study was the patient's lack of informed consent. None of the patients were told they had syphilis,

© Springer Nature Switzerland AG 2020
G. L. Hall, *Patient-Centered Clinical Care for African Americans*,
https://doi.org/10.1007/978-3-030-26418-5_2

instead they were told they had "bad blood" that required ongoing monitoring. In exchange for taking part in the study, the men received free medical exams, free meals, and burial insurance. Many physicians, including African Americans, and national physician societies, fully supported the study.

During the study, researchers not only allowed the disease to progress but actively blocked the men from receiving curable treatment, not just from the study physicians but also from other community physicians. The researchers implemented a coordinated effort … a verified conspiracy, with area physicians and hospitals to actively block treatment for the study participants if they presented elsewhere for care. Needless to say, this endeavor required the widespread dissemination of personal health information across an entire region and involving hundreds of people. The names and a stigmatizing diagnosis were circulated widely, and in a way that the patient would not know [2]. The fact that nearly 400 African American men were denied effective treatment for syphilis without their knowledge or consent so that researchers could document the natural history of the disease, stands as a singular event that granularly validates the mistrust African Americans have against the medical establishment.

It wasn't until 1972, when a news article reported the details of the study, that a government review panel finally halted it. The Tuskegee Health Benefit Program was established as a settlement for the class action suit brought against the United States which agreed to pay all medical and burial expenses for the subjects involved, with added support for their families. During the course of the study, 40 wives contracted the disease, and 19 children were born with congenital syphilis. Many credit the Tuskegee Syphilis Study as the primary reason informed consent regulations exist today. Unfortunately for many African Americans, the study is a validated reason to not trust doctors, public health, medical research, or the healthcare system.

Some might argue that with the passage of time and lower health literacy among some African Americans, the Tuskegee Syphilis Study is merely a historical footnote for most African Americans. A study done at Johns Hopkins looked at awareness of the Tuskegee Syphilis Study and found an overwhelming number of African Americans (81%) were aware of the study and outcomes, while only 28% of European Americans had knowledge of the study [5]. Another study demonstrated widespread misinformation as it relates to the Tuskegee study, but the authors still concluded that the study had tremendous "social power" [6]. With widespread knowledge of this government-sanctioned and funded study among African Americans, mentioning the study as a way to stimulate discussion, and build trust, is a preferable approach to ignoring its existence.

2.2   Other Examples of Abuse

While the Tuskegee Syphilis Study is a "classic example" of abuse based purely on race, unfortunately the American experience has many more examples of why African Americans mistrust the medical community.

From African American's earliest days in this country, abuse based on race was commonplace. Slaves were frequently used as subjects for dissection, surgical experimentation, and medical testing. J. Marion Sims, the so-called father of modern gynecology, perfected many of his surgical techniques on un-anaesthetized slave girls [7–9]. Stories of doctors kidnapping and killing southern blacks for experimentation consistently appear in literature throughout American history [10] (see Harriet Washington's book "Medical Apartheid" for a detailed review of this horrendous history).

As Vanesa Northington Gamble put in her article "Under the Shadow of Tuskegee: African Americans and Health Care" tales of "medical student," grave robbers recount the exploitation of southern African Americans as their deceased family members would be stolen and sent to northern medical schools for anatomy dissection [10]. Dr. Gamble writes:

> These historical examples clearly demonstrate that African Americans' distrust of the medical profession has a longer history than the public revelations of the Tuskegee Syphilis Study. There is a collective memory among African Americans about their exploitation by the medical establishment. [11]

2.3   Differences in Trust

Chanita Hughes Halbert published a study in Journal of the American Medical Association (JAMA) in 2006 looking at racial differences in trust in healthcare providers. Her study of almost one thousand European American and African American patients found that "compared with European Americans, African Americans were most likely to report low trust in healthcare providers" [1].

> Trust has been described as an expectation that medical care providers (physicians, nurses, and others) will act in ways that demonstrate that the patient's interests are a priority. Trust is a multidimensional construct that includes perceptions of the health care provider's technical ability, interpersonal skills, and the extent to which the patient perceives that his or her welfare is placed above other considerations. Trust is an important determinant of adherence to treatment and screening recommendations and the length and quality of relationships with health care providers. [1]

Fortunately, the level of trust a patient has for any specific provider is not stagnant, it can be earned. Increased exposure to providers in general, and to the same provider in specific, has been shown to improve trust.

Studies have also shown that *racial concordance* positively impacts the level of trust for a same race patient [12]. In simpler terms, African American patients are initially more trustful of African American providers. Those non-African American providers can, and do, achieve high levels of trust with African American patients, but doing so usually takes a little more effort.

2.4   Trust Improves Health Outcomes

In 1979 Russell Caterinicchio published what is believed to be the first study attempting to measure trust in patients for their physician and its impact on outcomes [13]. They made a clear distinction between trust and satisfaction, with trust as a condition that characterizes the present and future relationship and satisfaction characterizing past encounters and outcomes. Subsequent studies have confirmed and validated what providers suspected: there is a one-to-one correlation with trust in providers and self-rated health, therapeutic response, adherence to treatments, and decreased cost of care [14].

Conversely the lack of trust in providers has been associated with lower rates of care-seeking, preventative services, surgical treatment, and overall care. In David Thom's article "Measuring Trust in Physicians When Assessing Quality of Care," "increasing trust generally falls into the categories of competency, communication, caring, honesty, and partnering [15]." He cites prior studies that listed the following components of a trusting relationship:

1. Greater perceived mutual interests
2. Clear communication
3. A history of fulfilled trust
4. Less perceived difference in power with the person being trusted
5. Acceptance of personal disclosures
6. An expectation of a longer-term relationship

African American providers have a distinct advantage over others in the level of trust at the very beginning of their provider-patient relationship because of their mutual cultural history. As African Americans, there is clearly a perception of comparable mutual interests, as well as a less perceived difference in power. Clearer communication may also come from the better translation of complicated medical concepts into terms and analogies that have a similar cultural basis in the African American experience.

Thom goes on to explain how a provider can achieve these components of trust:

> All of these associations suggest approaches that would be expected to increase patient trust, such as emphasizing mutual interests (the patient's health); checking patients' understanding of communication; taking opportunities to fulfill trust (phoning with test results); reducing power differences (sharing information); responding to patients' self-disclosures in a supportive and nonjudgmental way; and promoting continuity of care. [15]

There are also differences in the acceptance of personal disclosures across racial lines with African Americans physicians being more tolerant of disclosures that may be more pervasive in their social community. The disclosure that a patient was raised in a single-parent family and has "no idea" what medical problems their father has may flow more smoothly to an African American provider who would be perceived as having a higher likelihood of not stigmatizing that history.

African American patients are also generally on guard for biases whether conscious or unconscious. More formally known as explicit and implicit biases, researchers have looked at the impact bias can have on the quality of patient encounters. Implicit biases are subconscious, whereas explicit biases are those that the practitioner is fully aware of. Providers may have an explicit bias against patients that were child molesters (as one extreme example) or against patients that are unemployed and presumably not seeking work (a subtler example). When a provider has an explicit bias, one that they admit to themselves and others, they typically work to minimize the effect of the bias on their quality of care. What is presumed is the provider's ability to work through those acknowledged explicit biases and still work for the full benefit of the patient.

Implicit biases are attitudes and stereotypes that impact our care delivery, discussion, and decisions in an unconscious manner. As noted by the Kirwan Institute for the Study of Race and Ethnicity at The Ohio State University, "implicit biases are pervasive. Everyone possesses them, even people with avowed commitments to impartiality such as judges." They go on to propose that "the implicit associations we hold do not necessarily align with our declared beliefs or even reflect stances we would explicitly endorse [16]." So many of us have no idea what our implicit biases may be … what is important is to accept that they exist and to work to get a better understanding for how they impact the care we provide.

In the "Medscape Internist Lifestyle Report 2017," Carol Peckham looked at internist's admitted explicit biases "toward specific types or groups of patients" and found wide differences between racial groups with 75% of Japanese internists admitting bias versus 29% of Asian (non-Indian) physicians [17]. A little over half (54%) of African American internists admitted to patient biases. Being biased against patients with emotional problems led the list, and over half of internists reported this issue. Physicians also reported biases toward or against patients that were overweight, have low intelligence, speak a different language, lack insurance, have low income, are older, have a different race, are physically unattractive, or are from a different gender (in decreasing occurrence). Providers were clearly biased to the benefit of older patients, but the other biases listed were generally negative or mixed outcome biases. These biases are not mutually exclusive. If a negatively biased providers see a poor, under-educated, older, obese, African American woman without insurance, they have a significant number of conscious biases impacting their care. There were also distinct gender differences with men having more biases than woman across the board. The study further examined if the physician bias actually impacted care delivery, and almost one in five providers (18%) admitted that their bias did impact the quality of their care.

Generally these biases are positive toward European American patients and negative toward African American patients as a study by Oliver et al. demonstrated at the University of Virginia [18]. They found providers explicitly preferred European Americans to African Americans with "significantly higher feelings of warmth toward (European Americans)" and also found that European American patients were "more medically cooperative than African Americans." The study found no significant difference in the quality of care between the racial groups. These biases can be consciously counteracted, and admitting the existence of biases is the critical first step in canceling its effect on medical care.

A study done at Johns Hopkins by Lisa Cooper and colleagues found that primary care physicians who hold unconscious racial biases tend to dominate conversations with African American patients during routine visits, paying less attention to patients' social and emotional needs, and making these patients feel less involved in decision-making related to their health [19]. These patients also reported reduced trust in their doctors, less respectful treatment, and a lower likelihood of recommending the physician to a friend.

Louis Penner and colleagues studied the impact bias has on medical interactions with African American patients and found that implicit biases impacted perceptions more dramatically than explicit biases and that these subtly biased behaviors were perceived as more deceitful than overt explicit bias [17]:

> Whereas people are aware of their overt and deliberative (e.g., verbal) behaviors, which relate to explicit measures of their attitudes, they may be unaware of their subtly biased and

spontaneous (e.g., nonverbal) behaviors, which relate to implicit measures. As targets of these behaviors, however, (African Americans) and members of other disadvantaged groups attend closely to these subtly biased behaviors, which critically shape their impressions of intergroup interactions. [20]

Coming to recognize implicit bias and its impact on medical decision-making, and then sensitizing providers regarding their ability to correct for these covert biases, is an important step in providing equitable care. Correcting for biases eliminates unspoken barriers to trust.

A study by L. Ebony Boulware, in addition to confirming much lower levels of trust in African American patients, also found elevated concerns about personal privacy and the potential for harmful experimentation [21]. This is a culturally driven privacy concern based on historical trust violations suffered by African Americans. While HIPPA laws protect everyone's health information, a patient may not be as aware of these restrictions on sharing patients' information. Making a point of emphasizing the privacy of their information and your discussions, as well as affirming the absence of experimentation, can go a long way to reassuring a skeptical patient.

With the earnest goal of providing high-quality comprehensive care, many "review-of-system"-type questions done routinely at an initial visit may strike some patients as overly probing and bordering on obtrusive. Imagine coming in for a hip replacement and having questions regarding a history of erection problems, depression, or prior abortions. While some may view these questions as consistent with being thorough, others could easily see them as invasive, and not pertinent.

When the provider is aware of the inclination on the part of the patient to "wonder" why they are asking unrelated health problems, it is advisable to explain the rationale or simply skip sensitive review-of-system questions that are not clearly pertinent to the diagnosis or discussion at hand until a more trusting rapport can be established.

Trust can be developed over time, but this requires continuity and is negatively impacted by urban clinic environments that have high physician turnover or have predominant physician extenders that may limit access to the primary care provider. A study by Mark Doescher and colleagues found a disparity in the trust for healthcare providers, and additionally found that low trust levels sink lower when on subsequent visits physician continuity was not preserved [22].

Although this seems obvious, spending time with patients is an easy approach to establishing trust. Fiscella and colleagues measured patient trust against the time spent with a patient and found a one-to-one correlation: the more time spent led to more perceived trust on the part of the patient [23].

Paul Duberstein et al. looked specifically at what impacts patients "satisfaction" with doctors and found that "openness" was associated with a much higher satisfaction rating that any of the other variables [24]. Openness, or a tendency toward self-revelations, as a way to connect, simply decreases the perceived barriers between patient and provider. The humanizing effects of discussing the provider's personal vulnerabilities while developing a relationship with a patient goes a long way to build trust. The patient has come to present their personal or medical deficiencies, and without some small degree of disclosure on the provider's part, the relationship seems overly one-sided. Divulging something as simple as "I'm terrible at typing on computers" will go far to diffuse some patients who may feel too large a difference in perceived power and stance. Openness facilitates the transfer of historically pertinent information that could be vital to the accurate diagnosis and treatment of many patients.

When it comes to African Americans specifically, Myra Sabir and Karl Pillemer looked at ways to gain the trust of older African Americans and improve their involvement with research [25]. In their study "An intensely sympathetic aware-ness: Experiential similarity and cultural norms as means for gaining older African Americans' trust of scientific research," they applied trust building techniques with great success. By specifically honoring and reinforcing older African Americans' worth and dignity through "high touch hospitality" measures, they were able to enlist and retain a significantly higher level of participation than the norm. Put sim-ply, they complimented their patients, and the patients appreciated their compli-ments. The researchers also race-matched the primary researcher with the subjects. In addition to preserving the continuity of the primary researcher from week to week, they also sent birthday and holiday cards, and finally, they took advantage of experiential similarities as a way to bond.

Because of the struggles of many African Americans, confessing a degree of struggle in your own life not only shows openness but a vulnerability that can lead to a trusting connection. By "explicitly emphasizing similarities," they were able to break down barriers to trust and empathy. While some patients are emboldened by an invincibly intelligent and successful physician, African Americans identify more with professionals they can identify with ... one that struggled and persisted. While a majority patient would likely prefer a physician who has succeeded in all they did, minority patients look to connect through a similar redemptive experience, and the honesty to share that experience.

Applying these shared experience measures might be a challenge for a 25-year-old European American suburban male nurse practitioner ... someone who may not have experienced much up until that point in his life. But a viable alternative is to talk about family members who the listener can identify with, like a father or grandmother who had struggles. Another approach is to concentrate on experiences that "reach the threshold of 'meaningful' for all persons," like survival, perseverance, and self-assurance. Confessing that you need to look up specific details of some more rare medical conditions or that you have family dynamics that can be stressful at times can add to your overall relatability.

2.5   Show Competence

One final, yet critical, approach to establishing a trust or unified rapport is to show competence in your environment, demeanor, and your examination. Showing competence is a simple yet undeniable aspect of assuming the care of African American patients. All patients want to know that their physician is competent, but African Americans may need a little more obvious evidence.

This air of competence begins with the environment of the office. Is it clean? Is there objective evidence of competence? Having diplomas and photos demonstrating a high level of competence can improve the early confidence a patient may place in the provider. Letting the patient know where you went to school, or that you have connections with the mayor or local official, for example, may also boost early confidence.

How have the staff presented themselves? What are the other patients in the waiting room saying about the provider? Answering the phone respectfully, seeing the patient in a timely fashion, and calling the patient with laboratory results or in response to an inquiry all show fundamental interpersonal competence that is both noticed and appreciated by the patient. Your respect for "patients" in general is critically important, and it shows in your environment of care. Due to racial concordance satisfaction outcomes, if your practice has a significant African American population (and you are not African American), it would be beneficial to have staff members that reflect that population.

After a fruitful discussion and thorough history has been obtained, a thoughtful and respectful physical examination can do much to clarify the awareness of your competence. Abraham Verghese in his article "The Bedside Evaluation: Ritual and Reason" in the *Annals of Internal Medicine*, discusses the art, mastery, and connection forged by the physical exam … as well as potential pitfalls [26].

> By giving permission to be examined, the patient affirms the physician's connection with and commitment to the patient—a transformation of both roles is occurring. The patient accords authority to the physician, but it is a gift of authority that many physicians take for granted. The years of study and a busy practice may get in the physician's way of seeing the therapeutic authority from a patient's standpoint. Conversely, the patient's cultural

background might contradict or supersede the authority the physician has presumed. The inherent power imbalance in the examination clearly has the potential to harm. Although the presence of a chaperone, parent, or nurse is an attempt to address these issues, the evaluation can still feel like a violation if not done gently, with careful attention to draping, patient modesty, and comfort. In certain cultures, the ritual could be viewed as a serious breach of trust.

We all fundamentally understand that a patient has the right to refuse certain aspects of the physical exam without retribution. Asking permission for the right to examine certain sensitive areas of the body is completely appropriate, and in some cases, expected. This discussion is best approached during the historical aspect of the visit. For example, many female patients may not intuitively understand why a pelvic exam may be necessary if they only presented with urinary tract symptoms. Explaining the rationale early in the visit can do much to allay confusion.

Once permission to perform a detailed and thoughtful exam has been granted, the examination "ritual" as Dr. Verghese describes is a key part of "conveying a symbolic centering of attention on the body as a locus of personhood as well as disease." The patient, in a very literal sense, exposes themselves both figuratively and literally to us. This vulnerable and sacred connection between clinician and patient should be treated by both parties as the ultimate demonstration of a sober offering and receiving of trust.

Do not destroy the sanctity or ritual of the clinician's touch by wearing gloves inappropriately. Competence also means following accepted guidelines. OSHA requirements are clear: gloves should be used during all patient-care activities that may involve exposure to blood and all other body fluids [27]. Yet many younger clinicians have begun to wear gloves throughout a physical exam that does not involve bodily fluids. Clinicians that wear gloves according to current guidelines will be compared to the "constant" glove-wearers and confuse patients as to which is actually appropriate. Many African Americans will assume the glove-wearers "don't want to touch them" when compared to physicians they trust that follow guidelines. Establishing a trusting clinician-patient relationship is much easier in the presence of a healing, comforting, or reassuring touch.

Obtain the trust of your patients. Once trust is given and respectfully accepted, it should be valued and revered as the greatest gift a patient could give to their provider.

Establishing Trust

1. Explore ways to discover *implicit biases* and work to minimize their impact on clinical encounters.
2. *Invest time:* set aside slightly more time early on in the provider-patient relationship.
3. Make *affirming comments* and compliments.
4. Make *personal disclosures.*
5. *Emphasize your similarities* with the patient.
6. *Acknowledge the unequal care* history but affirm equal care going forward.
7. *Reserve "sensitive" historical questions* for issues that are specifically related to the presenting condition.
8. Show *competence.*
9. Perform a thoughtful and respectful *physical exam.*
10. *Touch* your patients.

References

1. Halbert C, Armstrong K, Gandy O, Shaker B. Racial differences in trust in health care providers. Arch Intern Med. 2006;166(8):896–901.
2. Blendon RJ, Buhr T, Cassidy EF, et al. Disparities in physician care: experiences and perceptions of a multi-ethnic America. Health Aff (Millwood). 2008;27(2):507–17.
3. Brawley O. The study of untreated syphilis in the negro male. Int J Ratiat Oncol Biol Phys. 1998;40(1):5–8.
4. U.S. Public Health Service Syphilis Study at Tuskegee. Centers for Disease Control and Prevention. https://www.cdc.gov/tuskegee/index.html.
5. Shavers V, Lynch C, Burmeister L. Knowledge of the Tuskegee study and its impact on the willingness to participate in medical research studies. J Natl Med Assoc. 2000;92(12):563–72.
6. Green B, Li L, Morris J, Gluzman R, Davis J, Wang M, Katz R. Detailed knowledge of the Tuskegee syphilis study: who knows what? A framework for health promotion strategies. Health Educ Behav. 2011;38(6):629–36.
7. Ojanuga D. The medical ethics of the "father of gynaecology", Dr J Marion Sims. J Med Thics. 1993;19(1):28–31.
8. Spettel S, White MD. The portrayal of J. Marion Sims' controversial legacy. J Urol. 2011;185(6):2424–7.
9. Sartin JS. J. Marion Sims, the father of gynecology: hero or villain? South Med J. 2004;97(5):500–5.
10. Washington H. Medical apartheid: the dark history of medical experimentation on black Americans from colonial times to the present. 1st ed. Harlem Moon: Doubleday; 2006.

11. Gamble V. Under the shadow of Tuskegee: African Americans and health care. Am J Public Health. 1997;87(11):1773–8.
12. Blanchard J, Nayar BA, Lurie N. Patient-provider and patient-staff racial concordance and perceptions of mistreatment in the healthcare setting. J Gen Intern Med. 2007;22(8):1184–9.
13. Caterinicchio RP. Testing plausible path models of interpersonal trust in patient-physician treatment relationships. Soc Sci Med Part A. 1979;13:81–99.
14. Cuffee YL, Hargraves JL, Rosal M. Reported racial discrimination, trust in physicians, and medication adherence among inner-city African Americans with hypertension. Am J Public Health. 2013;103(11):e55–62.
15. Thom D, Hall M, Pawlson G. Measuring patients' trust in physicians when assessing quality of care. Health Aff (Millwood). 2004;23(4):124–32.
16. Kirwan Institute for the Study of Race and Ethnicity. http://kirwaninstitute.osu.edu/.
17. Peckham C. Medscape lifestyle report 2017. Race and ethnicity, bias and burnout. https://www.medscape.com/features/slideshow/lifestyle/2017/overview.
18. Oliver M, Wells K, Joy-Gaba J, Hawkins C, Nosek B. Do physcians' implicit views of African Americans affect clinical decision making? J Am Board Fam Med. 2014;27(2):177–88.
19. Cooper L, Roter D, Carson K, Beach M, Sabin J, Greenwald A, Inui T. The associations of clinicians' implicit attitudes about race with medical visit communication and patient ratings of interpersonal care. Am J Public Health. 2012;102(5):979–87.
20. Penner L, Dovidio J, West T, Gaertner S, Albrecht T, Daily R, Markova T. Aversive racism and medical interactions with black patients: a field study. J Exp Soc Psychol. 2010;46(2):436–40.
21. Boulware L, Cooper L, Ratner L, LaVeist T, Powe N. Race and trust in the health care system. Public Health Rep. 2003;118(4):358–65. https://www.ncbi.nlm.nih.gov/pmc/articles/PMC1497554/pdf/12815085.pdf.
22. Doescher M, Saver B, Fiscella K, Franks P. Preventive care: does continuity count? J Gen Intern Med. 2004;19(6):632–7.
23. Fiscella K, Meldrum S, Franks P, Shields C, Duberstein P, McDaniel S, Epstein R. Patient trust: is it related to patient-centered behavior of primary care physicians? Med Care. 2004;42(11):1049–55.
24. Duberstein P, Meldrum S, Fiscella K, Shields C, Epstein R. Influences on patients' ratings of physicians: physicians demographics and personality. Patient Educ Couns. 2007;65(2):270–4.
25. Sabir M, Pillemer K. An intensely sympathetic awareness: experiential similarity and cultural norms as means for gaining older African Americans' trust of scientific research. J Aging Stud. 2014;29:142–9.
26. Verghese A, Brady E, Kapur C, Horwitz R. The bedside evaluation: ritual and reason. Ann Intern Med. 2011;155(8):550–3.
27. World Health Organization. Glove use information leaflet. http://www.who.int/gpsc/5may/Glove_Use_Information_Leaflet.pdf.

Delivering Consistent and Equitable Healthcare

3

Being consistent and equitable in your care of African Americans is critical and has been key to decreasing a number of health disparities. Consistency (doing the same thing the same way each time) and equity (providing fair and impartial treatment) can at times be at odds because technically, they are not the same. What modern healthcare strives to do is be more consistent across populations, and this attempt at consistency frequently fails due to variability in access, insurance coverage, provider idiosyncrasies, and patient need. African Americans statistically have worse access and get less clinical interventions in many cancers and chronic diseases [1]. Providing better care to African American patients will require more insight into why their care is currently inferior, and a closer look at what has worked to decrease health disparities in this population.

Modern protocols instituted and mandated at hospitals across the country have seen disparities shrink when these protocols are consistently applied across populations for chest pain, pneumonia, or stroke symptoms, for example [2–6]. The reality is that if true wide-spread consistency were achieved, disparities in healthcare would still exist because a consistent approach across different patient populations will invariably lead to unequal outcomes. Screening a European American population for sickle cell anemia or an African American population for cystic fibrosis would be a waste of financial resources. Providers are well aware of "differences" in an approach to care, or a predilection for occurrence for many disorders between patient populations and/or gene pools. Clinicians learned of a greatly increased risk for breast cancer or colon cancer in Ashkenazi Jews [7, 8], for example, and with increased research and data analysis, a number of differences and idiosyncrasies have been discovered relating to the care and treatment of African American

© Springer Nature Switzerland AG 2020
G. L. Hall, *Patient-Centered Clinical Care for African Americans*,
https://doi.org/10.1007/978-3-030-26418-5_3

patients as well. A reasonable approach would dictate that we first educate ourselves about these differences, and then apply nuanced clinical care when appropriate.

The concept of health equity is fundamental in all of medicine. Provide the medical care that the patient requires … no more and no less. The time that we spend learning about the nuances of diseases in different settings, and expecting variable outcomes in different populations, prepares us for competent care in our clinical practice.

Providing equitable care means all patients would get the care and screening they "need." Using this logic, only smokers would get smoking cessation counseling, not everyone. Patient populations known to get aggressive versions of certain disorders would receive more stringent screening than other populations (i.e., Kawasaki disease in Asian and Pacific Islanders or prostate cancer in African American males). Because of the challenges of unequal care in America, striving for improved widespread consistency is still a goal worth pursuing and will continue to shrink disparities because of the many genetic and physiologic similarities across populations. But health equity is the true ultimate healthcare goal: medical care tailored specifically to the patient.

The US Agency for Healthcare Research and Quality presents an annual National Healthcare Quality and Disparities Report which tracks health outcomes and the progress for eliminating disparities [9]. Year after year disparities based on race, income, and other factors are tracked by clinical measures. Outcomes such as time to electrocardiogram after presentation with chest pain, or patient satisfaction with physician communication, are measured and reported. Hospital scores are publically presented, and benchmarks set for comparison. Significant outliers are financially impacted. By having protocols for critical presentations, the process of deciding who gets what medical tests and when has been moved from the clinician to a "knee-jerk" process mediated by presentation. While this is seen by some to negatively impact the "art" of medicine (and it unquestionably does in some circumstances), it has had a great impact in decreasing a host of racial and gender disparities based on how a person presents.

Our responsibility as clinicians is to provide equitable care regardless of insurance, financial resources, or access. Because we are constantly presented with barriers to equitable care in the form of medication formularies, prior authorizations for studies, patients ability to comply with an order, and our own biases, we frequently acquiesce and settle for the less-than-ideal alternative. A patient with "good insurance" presenting with a very high cholesterol can initially get the best statin medication to lower their cholesterol to target, while a "managed care insurance" patient may have to use a less efficacious statin drug first, fail to reach their goal, and then progress to the "better" drug we would have chosen without being "managed." While progressing through this "managed care" process will result in more affordable care, and may occasionally reveal success with a first line statin, prolonging the path to successful cholesterol lowering will frustrate many patients, jeopardize ongoing compliance due to patients questioning our competence, prolong cardiovascular risk exposure, and impede our ability to reach target controls in our patient populations.

As these small impedances to proper care accumulate, foundational barriers are formed that comprise many of the health disparities based on socioeconomic status. When seeing poor patients, we have come to expect that some of our initial choices for medications will not get covered, or a radiologic study approved, and we adjust our care to work around these barriers (whether perceived or real). If we order an MRI of the head for a patient with severe headaches, we generally will see that order denied. After the first few denials, we begin to anticipate the denial and follow the next most appropriate course without first getting the denial. If we see this pattern with a specific insurance, we adjust our orders in response. As these stumbling blocks continue, we begin to categorize the barriers we see based on insurance, ability to pay, access, etc.

With African Americans comprising a higher percentage of the poor (20% for African Americans vs. 8% for European Americans) [10], some providers will categorize all African Americans as poor, and when they see an African American, they "anticipate" the more stringent insurance issues normally seen with the poor. Those adjustments based on anticipated barriers are followed, and the inferior outcomes associated with low income become a barrier to the 80% of African Americans that live above the poverty level. The adjustments that providers make are simply made as an approach to a complex and ever-changing set of clinical rules and restrictions. But put simply, the dynamics and disadvantages of poor patients' care place an additional burden on the care of some non-poor African Americans. These health disparities extend to outpatient rehabilitation therapy referrals which, again, are typically not easily approved in a "managed care" environment [11]. There was a "reduced likelihood of an office-based therapy visit for (African) Americans with arthritis when controlled for income, insurance, and education," a study by Sandstrom and Bruns published in the Journal of Racial and Ethnic Health Disparities [12]. This "stereotyping" by healthcare providers contributes to the disparate treatment plans seen when comparing racial outcomes. The preconceptions regarding a particular patients' tendency to follow through with an order, or an insurance preference to approve an order, or the effectiveness of a protocol in a particular racial population, are merely the clinicians' attempt to simplify a complicated set of conflicting inter-actions. Joseph Metancourt wrote about this stereotyping phenomenon:

> This is a normal, functional, adaptive, cognitive process that is automatic, and usually cen-ters on characteristics that manifest visually, such as race, gender, and age. Interestingly, we tend to activate stereotypes most when we are stressed, multitasking, and under the time pressure—the hallmarks of the clinical encounter.
>
> For example, many medical students and residents are often trained—and minorities cared for—in academic health centers or public hospitals located in socioeconomically disadvantaged areas. As a result, doctors may begin to equate certain races and ethnicities with specific health beliefs and behaviors (i.e., "these patients" engage in risky behaviors, or "those patients" tend to be noncompliant) that are more associated with the social envi-ronment (e.g., poverty) than patient's racial/ethnic background or cultural traditions. This stereotyping is a natural and expected—but no less dangerous—phenomenon that may affect the way doctors make decisions and offer specific interventions to different patients based on their race or ethnicity. [13]

The stereotyping, confounding, and preconception-forming behavior impacts clinical decision-making to the detriment of African Americans. Specialist referrals [14], advanced treatments for cancer [15], rheumatological condition chemothera-pies [16], and other "higher end" interventions that represent an escalation of care are all decreased in African Americans independent of socioeconomic status [17]. To be clear, these interventions represent clinician-written orders not impacted by patient condition or responsibility. The prospect of disentangling the confounding of race, socioeconomic status, and other preconceptions in African Americans can lead to significantly improved care.

With African Americans tending to live where African American's live, com-munity barriers to care also impact our ability to deliver consistent and equitable care. The most recent census data show that in the United States, 60% of African Americans live in only six states, and over half live in southern states where quality care outcomes are inferior [18] (Fig. 3.1).

"Hospital care for (African American) patients in the United States is remark-ably concentrated in a small percentage of hospitals" studies have confirmed [19]. The 5% of hospitals with the highest volume of African American patients care for nearly half of all elderly black patients.

Studies have also shown that patients without access to primary care providers have higher emergency services utilization. Curiously, in one study of emergency department use among African American HMO enrollees, they found a persis-tently higher use of the emergency department in African Americans even when they reported having a primary care provider [20]. The same study also found these

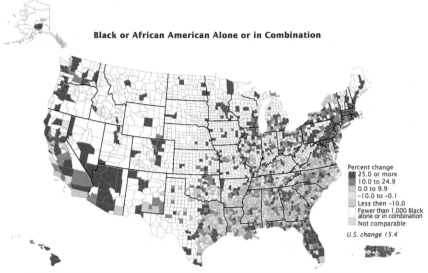

Black or African American Alone or in Combination

Percent change
- 25.0 or more
- 10.0 to 24.9
- 0.0 to 9.9
- −10.0 to −0.1
- Less then −10.0
- Fewer than 1,000 Black alone or in combination
- Not comparable

U.S. change 15.4

Sources: U.S. Census Bureau, *Census 2000 Redistricting Data (Public Law 94-171) Summary File*, Table PL1; and *2010 Census Redistricting Data (Public Law 94-171) Summary File*, Table P1.

Fig. 3.1 US African American population density (US Census Bureau). https://www.census.gov/prod/cen2010/briefs/c2010br-06.pdf

trends "after controlling for sociodemographic differences." The researchers supposed that the increased use of emergency services, even in the face of presumed primary care access, was likely driven by "dissatisfaction with a usual source of care, long waits to schedule appointments, ... belief in the urgency of the condition and the convenience of the emergency room [20]." This increased use of emergency services can stretch resources and impact access for all patients.

Emergency medical care for many in African American communities may actually start in an ambulance on the way to a hospital. Hospitals in high African American populated regions are more likely to be on "ambulance diversion" where the emergency services are temporarily closed to ambulance traffic due to overcrowding or a lack of other resources at the hospital (personnel and/or hospital beds) [21]. These diversions delay emergency treatment (intubations, surgeries, catheterizations), medical interventions (antibiotics for sepsis, pharmaceutical cardioversions), and many other diagnostic and lifesaving interventions. Numerous studies have shown the negative impact these delays in care have on clinical outcomes. Diversions were "associated with poorer access to cardiac technology, lower probability of receiving revascularization, and worse long-term mortality outcomes," a study in California reported [21]. Shen and Hsia, the authors of the study, found that racial disparities do exist and "(African American) patients are more likely to be diverted than (European American) patients because the ED closest to them is more likely to be on diversion [21]." In another study Hsia and colleagues found that in California, "hospitals serving minorities were more likely to divert, even when controlling for hospital ownership, emergency department capacity, and other hospital-level demographic and structural factors" [22]. Having to be diverted to another hospital will definitely impact care in terms of medical history and records access, provider familiarity, timeliness of care, and countless other factors.

Once at a hospital, African Americans still have worse outcomes. Karen Joynt at the Department of Health Policy and Management at the Harvard School of Public Health looked at the 30-day readmission rate for all fee-for-service Medicare recipients for a 3-year period [13]. Her examination of over 3 million discharges found a number of adverse quality outcomes based purely on race. She found a trend among *minority-serving hospitals*, which were defined as hospitals in the "highest decile (10%) of proportion of (African American) patients … while the other 90% of hospitals were categorized as nonminority-serving":

> At minority-serving hospitals, on average, 37% of patients were (African American), compared with 1.4% of patients at non-minority-serving hospitals. Minority-serving hospitals were more often large, public or for-profit hospitals. Seventy percent of the minority-serving hospitals were located in the south, compared with 35% of the non-minority-serving hospitals. Minority-serving hospitals were more often teaching hospitals, and served a higher proportion of Medicaid patients… Minority-serving hospitals had fewer nurses per 1000 patient-days, and had somewhat lower performance on HQA measures. Length of stay was greater at minority-serving hospitals for each condition. [13]

Across the board, African American patients were much more likely to be admitted to a minority-serving hospital (40% chance versus a 1.4% chance for whites) and had a 13% higher odds of all-cause 30-day readmission than European Americans. They also found that "(European American) patients at nonminority serving hospitals consistently had the lowest odds of readmission, and (African American) patients at minority-serving hospitals (had) the highest." Interestingly, African American patients at nonminority-serving hospitals got care essentially equivalent to white patients at minority serving hospitals. Overall this analysis found that:

> … elderly (African American) patients had higher odds of 30-day readmission than (European American) patients for AMI, CHF, and pneumonia. These disparities were related to race itself as well as to the site where care was provided: (African American) patients had a 13% higher odds of readmission than (European American) patients, while patients discharged from minority-serving hospitals had a 23% higher odds of readmission than patients discharged from non-minority-serving hospitals. [23]

3.1   **African American Clinical Care Disparities**

The African American racial differences in outcomes while hospitalized are numerous and include:

- Increased mortality from acute respiratory failure from sepsis [24].
- Highest stroke mortality and morbidity [25].
- Less likely to receive thrombolytic treatment [26] at both primary stroke centers and non-primary stroke centers and less likely to be discharged on secondary prevention measures (including lipid-lowering medications) [25].
- Less likely to be on warfarin with atrial fibrillation [27].
- Lower physician-ordered cholesterol screens [28].
- Decreased use of pharmacotherapy for hyperlipidemia [28].
- Increased leg amputations [29]. African Americans "comprise 29% of patients undergoing a major lower extremity amputation, but only 12% of those undergoing an open surgical procedure and 10% of those undergoing an endovascular procedure for limb salvage" [30].
- Worse postoperative outcomes after pituitary brain surgery [31].
- Increased risk of complications and/or mortality following spine surgical or joint replacement procedures [32].
- Lower incidence of receiving trans-catheter aortic valve replacement for severe aortic stenosis [33].
- Lower rates of initiating hemodialysis with an AV fistula (the preferred approach) when controlled for insurance and despite being younger and having fewer comorbidities [34].
- Higher morbidity and mortality in inflammatory bowel diseases [35].
- Worse childhood asthma admissions with complications [36].
- Decreased use of Alzheimer disease pharmacotherapy [37].
- Decreased rates of diagnosis and treatment of depression with an antidepressant [38].
- Lower physician-ordered diet/nutrition counseling [28].
- Lower physician-ordered exercise counseling [28].

Cancer outcomes are also stunning with the worst outcomes in:

- Lung [39, 40]
- Liver [41]
- Colon [42]
- Ovarian [43]

- Endometrial [44]
- Breast [44]
- Prostate cancer [45]
- Head and neck cancer [46]
- Oropharyngeal cancer survival [47]
- Worst outcomes and less likely to undergo bone marrow transplant and get effective treatment (bortezomib) in multiple myeloma [48]

Also related to cancer outcomes, African Americans have:

- Greater myeloproliferative progression and complications [49]
- Increased complications from thyroid surgery [50] and worse outcomes from thyroid cancer [51]
- Lower incidence of partial nephrectomy for solitary renal masses ("better than total nephrectomy for limited size tumors") [52]

Many of these poor outcomes are at least partially driven by provider action ... or inaction. The dicey question is always "who is contributing to these disparities?". The uncomfortable answer is: we all contribute.

3.2 Variability in Our Care

Care approaches based on what an insurance allows, or an anticipated non-compliance, or a presumed poor outcome, result in unequal care. We assume that unequal care results in superior care for some and inferior care for others, but in the end, we all provide unequal care. If your favorite US president or most admired celebrity presented for medical care in your hospital, you would likely more closely review your clinical decisions. You would spend more time with the patient, order more labs and radiographic studies, and if needed, you would research every aspect of their presenting complaints. In a sense, they would get the best care you could provide. But keep in mind that providing everyone with that level of care is intensive, expensive, impractical, and unadvisable. So do not beat yourself up too badly for adding to health disparities!

But also do not delude yourself into thinking you provide consistent and equal care. By acknowledging that your care varies, you are actually taking the first critical step to decreasing disparities in your own practice. While some clinicians are quick to acknowledge obvious ongoing unequal care, others flatly reject the notion of unequal care ... particularly in America.

Let's put racial disparities' aside for a moment. My patients that smell badly do not get great care from me. Since I was a child, I always had a weak stomach in response to bad smells. When I walk into an exam room and the patient smells badly of urine or stool, or has very bad breath, I will be acutely aware of, and distracted by, the smell. I will proceed to get as brief a history as I can, do a somewhat distracted exam, and exit as quickly as possible without being overtly disrespectful. In my defense, I will try to compensate by doing more background research, documenting more thoroughly, and making follow-up phone calls to fill in the gaps caused by my weak stomach. These patients get less small talk, less history taking, and a faster exam. I provide different care to that population, and because I haven't learned to control my nasogastric reflexes, I cannot change the basics of the situation. Because I go out of my way to compensate for my weakness, I do not believe this population gets inferior care from me, but I know for sure that they do not get superior care. A good degree of my strength as a physician stem from my personal "connection" with the patient and my intuition of their strengths and weaknesses as sensed during my personal time with them. Being distracted by adverse smells, reroutes my thinking, impairs my intuition, and impacts my in-person care.

I assume most clinicians lack my odiferous weakness and have no problem with this aspect of patient care, but I am sure there are other similar examples that some providers could report. Try giving equal care and time to a mean and spiteful person, or a child rapist? During the recent opioid addiction epidemic, caregivers have been treating pregnant and new mothers with high systemic opioid levels in themselves and toxic levels in their baby's systems. The perceived irresponsibility of these situations tests provider's tolerance and ability to give complete and compassionate care to mothers that they perceive as abusive to their unborn or newly born child. In short, providers are offended by the irresponsibility of these mothers and have difficulty forging a warm caring relationship with them. In reality, a forgiving and trusting therapeutic relationship with these addicted patients is the first critical step to the success of their treatment, but many providers struggle with this concept and put forth a more punishing and judgmental demeanor. While these provider reactions are natural and understandable, they are also inefficient and therapeutically counterintuitive.

Delivering consistent and equitable care in a number of clinical scenarios takes education, self-awareness (biases and all), and practice. Realizing that your care frequently varies due to a number of conflicting and compounding variables is the only approach to ultimately minimizing their impact. Acknowledging that your African American patient is prone for worse clinical outcomes and proactively compensating and advocating on your patient's behalf will drive down the clinician-driven disparate outcomes we see.

Delivering Consistent and Equitable Care

- Understand that from a racial standpoint and across an array of parameters, African Americans receive the worst clinical care.
- Equitable care means providing interventions that are "needed" and appropriate for the patient.
- Sometimes clinician orders and directives are influenced by presumptions related to socioeconomic status, insurance coverage patterns, and patient idiosyncrasies.
- 60% of African Americans live in only six states, and over half live in southern states.
- Hospital care for African American patients in the United States is remarkably concentrated in a small percentage of hospitals. The 5% of hospitals with the highest volume of African American patients care for nearly half of all elderly African American patients
- African Americans tend to follow community-specific referral patterns and go to hospitals where they feel "welcome."
- Hospitals with more minority patients see increased ambulance divergence and emergency department closures that negatively impact quality and continuity of care.
- We all have biases … both explicit and implicit.
- We all provide variable care that is dependent on our biases. The key is to be more self-aware.

References

1. 2015 National Healthcare Quality and Disparities Report Chartbook on Health Care for Blacks. Rockville: Agency for Healthcare Research and Quality; 2016. AHRQ Pub. No 16-0015-1-EF.
2. Gomez MA, Anderson JL, Karagounis LA, Muhlestein JB, Mooers FB. An emergency department-based protocol for rapidly ruling out myocardial ischemia reduces hospital time and expense: results of a randomized study (ROMIO). J Am Coll Cardiol. 1996;28:25–33.
3. Pope JH, Aufderheide TP, Ruthazer R, Woolard RH, Feldman JA, Beshansky JR, Griffith JL, Selker HP. Missed diagnoses of acute cardiac ischemia in the emergency department. N Engl J Med. 2000;342:1163–70.
4. Six AJ, Backus BE, Kelder JC. Chest pain in the emergency room: value of the HEART score. Neth Heart J. 2008;16:191–6.
5. Grief SN, Loza JK. Guidelines for the evaluation and treatment of pneumonia. Prim Care. 2018;45(3):485–503. https://doi.org/10.1016/j.pop.2018.04.001.
6. Meschia JF, Bushnell C, Boden-Albala B, et al. Guidelines for the primary prevention of stroke: a statement for healthcare professionals from the American Heart Association/American Stroke Association. Stroke. 2014;45(12):3754–832.

7. Rinella ES, Shao Y, Yackowski L, et al. Genetic variants associated with breast cancer risk for Ashkenazi Jewish women with strong family histories but no identifiable BRCA1/2 mutation. Hum Genet. 2013;132(5):523–36.

8. Jasperson KW, Tuohy TM, Neklason DW, Burt RW. Hereditary and familial colon cancer. Gastroenerology. 2010;138960:2044–58.

9. 2017 National Healthcare Quality and Disparities Report. Retrieved from https://www.ahrq.gov/research/findings/nhqrdr/nhqdr17/index.html. 2018. Accessed 8 May 2019.

10. Poverty rate by race/ethnicity. Henry J Kaiser Family Foundation. https://www.kff.org/other/state-indicator/poverty-rate-by-raceethnicity/. Accessed 9 May 2019.

11. Carvalho E, Bettger JP, Goode AP. Insurance coverage, costs, and barriers to care for outpatient musculoskeletal therapy and rehabilitation services. N C Med J. 2017;78(5):312–4.

12. Sandstrom R, Bruns A. Disparities in access to outpatient rehabilitation therapy for African Americans with arthritis. J Racial Ethn Health Disparities. 2016;4(4):599–606.

13. Betancourt JR. Eliminating racial and ethnic disparities in health care: what is the role of academic medicine? Acad Med. 2006;81(9):788–92.

14. Simpson DR, Martínez ME, Gupta S, Hattangadi-Gluth J, Mell LK, Heestand G, et al. Racial disparity in consultation, treatment, and the impact on survival in metastatic colorectal cancer. JNCI: J Natl Cancer Inst. 2013;105(23):1814–20.

15. Murphy MM, Simons JP, Ng SC, Mcdade TP, Smith JK, Shah SA, et al. Racial differences in cancer specialist consultation, treatment, and outcomes for locoregional pancreatic adenocarcinoma. Ann Surg Oncol. 2009;16(11):2968–77. https://doi.org/10.1245/s10434-009-0656-5.

16. Katz JN, Barrett J, Liang MH, Kaplan H, Roberts W, Baron JA. Utilization of rheumatology physician services by the elderly. Am J Med. 1998;105(4):312–8.

17. LaVeist TA, Morgan A, Arthur M, Plantholt S, Rubinstein M. Physician referral patterns and race differences in receipt of coronary angiography. Health Serv Res. 2002;37(4):949–62.

18. Rastogi S, Johnson TT, Hoefell EM, Drewery MP Jr. The black population: 2010 – Census.gov. https://www.census.gov/prod/cen2010/briefs/c2010br-06.pdf. 2011. Accessed 8 May 2019.

19. Jha A, Orav E, Li Z, Epstein A. Concentration and quality of hospitals that care for elderly black patients. Arch Intern Med. 2007;167(11):1177–82.

20. Roby D, Nicholson G, Kominski G. African Americans in commercial HMO's more likely to delay prescription drugs and use emergency room. Policy Brief UCLA Cent Health Policy Res. 2009;(PB2009-7):1–12.

21. Shen Y, Hsia R. Do patients hospitalized in high-minority hospitals experience more diversion and poorer outcomes? A retrospective multivariate analysis of Medicare patients in California. BMJ Open. 2016;6(3):e010263.

22. Hsia R, Asch S, Weiss R, Zingmond D, Liang L, Han W, McCreath H, Sun B. California hospitals serving large minority populations were more likely than others to employ ambulance diversion. Health Aff (Millwood). 2012;31(8):1767–76.

23. Joynt K, Orav E, Jha A. Patient race, site of care, and 30-day readmission rates among elderly Americans. JAMA. 2011;305(7):675–81.

24. Bime C, Poongkunran C, Borgstrom M, Natt B, Desai H, Parthasarathy S, Garcia J. Racial differences in mortality from severe acute respiratory failure in the United States, 2008–2012. Ann Am Thorac. 2016;12(12):2184–9.

25. Cruz-Flores S, Biller J, Elkind M, et al. Racial-ethnic disparities in stroke care: the American experience: a statement for healthcare professionals from the American Heart Association/American Stroke Association. Stroke. 2011;42(7):2091–116.
26. Aparicio H, Carr B, Kasner S, Kallan M, Albright K, Kleindorfer D, Mullen M. Racial disparities in intravenous recombinant tissue plasminogen activator use persist at primary stroke centers. J Am Heart Assoc. 2015;4(10):e001877.
27. Amponsah M, Benjamin E, Magnani J. Atrial fibrillation and race – a contemporary review. Curr Cardiovasc Risk Rep. 2013;7(5):336. https://doi.org/10.1007/s12170-013-0327-8.
28. Willson M, Neumiller J, Sclar D, Robison L, Skaer T. Ethnicity/race, use of pharmacotherapy, scope of physician-ordered cholesterol screening, and provision of diet/nutrition or exercise counseling during office-based visits by patients with hyperlipidemia. Am J Cardiovasc Drugs. 2010;10(2):105–8.
29. Lefebvre K, Chevan J. The persistence of gender and racial disparities in vascular lower extremity amputation: an examination of HCUP-NIS data (2002–2011). Vasc Med. 2015;20(1):51–9.
30. Holman K, Henke P, Dimick J, Birkmeyer J. Racial disparities in the use of revascularization before leg amputation in medicare patients. J Vasc Surg. 2011;54(2):420–6, 426.e1.
31. Goljo E, Parasher A, Iloreta A, Shrivastava R, Govindaraj S. Racial, ethnic, and socioeconomic disparities in pituitary surgery outcomes. Laryngoscope. 2016;126(4):808–14.
32. Schoenfeld A, Tipirneni R, Nelson J, Carpenter J, Iwashyna T. The influence of race and ethnicity on complications and mortality after orthopedic surgery: a systematic review of the literature. Med Care. 2014;52(9):842–51.
33. Sleder A, Tackett S, Cerasale M, Mittal C, et al. Socioeconomic and racial disparities: a case-control study of patients receiving transcatheter aortic valva replacement for severe aortic stenosis. J Racial Ethn Health Disparities. 2017;4(6):1189–94.
34. Zarkowsky D, Arhuidese I, Hicks C, et al. Racial/ethnic disparities associated with initial hemodialysis access. JAMA Surg. 2005;150(6):529–36.
35. Nguyen G, Chong C, Chong R. National estimates of the burden of inflammatory bowel disease among racial and ethnic groups in the United States. J Crohns Colitis. 2014;8(4):288–95.
36. Woods E, Bhaumik U, Sommer S, et al. Community asthma initive to improve health outcomes and reduce disparities among children with asthma. MMWR Suppl. 2016;65(1):11–20.
37. Gilligan A, Malone D, Warholak T, Armstrong E. Racial and ethnic disparities in Alzheimer's disease pharmacotherapy exposure: an analysis across four state Medicaid populations. Am J Geriatr Pharmacother. 2012;10(5):303–12.
38. Sclar D, Robison L, Schmidt J, Bowen K, Castillo L, Oganov A. Diagnosis of depression and use of antidepressant pharmacotherapy among adults in the United States: does a disparity persist by ethnicity/race? Clin Drug Investig. 2012;32(2):139–44.
39. Sin M. Lung cancer disparities and African Americans. Public Health Nurs. 2017;34(4):359–62.
40. Ryan B. Lung cancer health disparities. Carcinogenesis. 2018;39(6):741–51.
41. Estevez J, Yang J, Leong J, et al. Clinical features associated with survival outcome in African American patients with hepatocellular carcinoma. Am J Gastroenterol. 2018;114:80. https://doi.org/10.1038/s41395-018-0261-y.
42. Busch E, Galanko J, Sandler R, Goel A, Keku T. Lifestyle factors, colorectal tumor methylation, and survival among African Americans and European Americans. Sci Rep. 2018;8:9470.

43. Collins Y, Holcomb K, Chapman-Davis E, Khabele D, Farley J. Gynecologic cancer dispari-
    ties: a report from the health disparities taskforce of the Society of Gynecologic Oncology.
    Gynecol Oncol. 2014;133(2):353–61.
44. DeSantis C, Fedewa S, Sauer A, et al. Breast cancer statistics, 2015: convergence of incidence
    rates between black and white women. CA Cancer J Clin. 2015;66:31–42.
45. Williams V, Awasthi S, Fink A, et al. African American men and prostate cancer-specific
    mortality: a competing risk analysis of a large institutional cohort, 1989–2015. Cancer Med.
    2018;7(5):2160–71.
46. Ragin C, Langevin S, Marzouk M, Grandis J, Taioli E. Determinants of head and neck cancer
    survival by race. Head Neck. 2011;33(8):1092–8.
47. Megwalu U, Ma Y. Racial disparities in oropharyngeal cancer survival. Oral Oncol.
    2017;65:33–7.
48. Fiala M, Wildes T. Racial disparities in treatment use for multiple myeloma. Cancer.
    2017;123(9):1590–6.
49. Khan I, Shergill A, Saraf S, et al. Outcome disparities in Caucasian and non-Caucasian patients
    with myeloproliferative neoplasms. Clin Lymphoma Myeloma Leuk. 2016;16(6):350–7.
50. Al-Qurayshi Z, Randolph G, Srivastav S, Aslam R, Friedlander P, Kandil E. Outcomes in
    thyroid surgery are affected by racial, economic, and healthcare system demographics.
    Laryngoscope. 2016;126(9):2194–9.
51. Megwalu U, Saini A. Racial disparities in papillary microcarcinoma survival. J Laryngol Otol.
    2017;131(1):83–7.
52. Kiechle J, Abouassaly R, Gross C, et al. Racial disparities in partial nephrectomy persist across
    hospital types: results from a population-based cohort. Urology. 2016;90:69–74.

Important Differences in Cardiovascular Care

4

There are a number of important differences in the care of African Americans that can substantially impact clinical outcomes including specific medication choices, disease control, and alternative clinical approaches. Applying these research-verified clinical management regimes can assuredly clear a more efficient path to clinical success and positively benefit outcomes.

African Americans are at a higher risk than European Americans for cardiovascular diseases as evidenced by their:

- 2-fold increased risk for stroke [1]
- 4-fold increased mortality from stroke [2]
- 2.5-fold increased risk for heart failure [1]
- 2-fold increased risk for sudden cardiac death [2]
- 1.5-fold increased risk for hypertension [2]
- 1.7-fold increased risk for diabetes [2]
- 4-fold increased risk for hospitalization due to uncontrolled diabetes [2]
- 2-fold increased risk for obesity [2]

4.1 Hypertension

The prevalence of hypertension in African Americans is the highest in the United States and one of the highest in the world [3], and there has been significant research pertaining to idiosyncrasies unique to this population. Hypertension has been associated with an increased risk of myocardial infarction, heart failure, stroke, and kidney disease. Beginning with a blood pressure at 115/75 mm Hg,

© Springer Nature Switzerland AG 2020
G. L. Hall, *Patient-Centered Clinical Care for African Americans*,
https://doi.org/10.1007/978-3-030-26418-5_4

an individual's risk of developing cardiovascular disease doubles with every additional rise of 20/10 mm Hg. Recent data regarding prevalence of hypertension using a threshold of 140/90 reveals a rate of 45% in African American men and 46% in African American women [4]. Other commonly accepted risk factors for hypertension include age, family history, obesity, individual and neighborhood socioeconomic status, and a number of lifestyle factors including activity level, diet, and tobacco use. Digging deeper into the causes of hypertension, Deborah Rohm Young and colleagues found that hypertension rates within African Americans did not vary significantly based on neighborhood socioeconomic status or progressive obesity [5].

> In this large, racially/ethnically and geographically diverse overweight and obese sample, we found that all racial and ethnic minorities, except Hispanics, had higher odds of diagnosed hypertension prevalence across all weight categories and neighborhood education levels compared with whites. In general, although tests for two-way interactions were significant, compared with whites, the magnitude of the odds of hypertension for each racial/ ethnic category compared with whites did not substantially vary based on overweight/obese weight category or neighborhood education category. Our results suggest that these factors may not explain the racial/ethnic disparities in hypertension prevalence compared with whites. [5]

The overwhelming evidence in this study curiously found that African Americans living in high socioeconomic neighborhoods and presumably making significantly higher income while having access to healthier foods and exercise opportunities still cannot escape a significantly increased hypertension risk. There must be a genetic predisposition.

Among the genetic differences getting much of the attention in hypertensive African Americans is the potential existence of a salt-sensitive gene that may make hypertension worse [6]. Jonathan Williams and colleagues looked specifically at a "lysine-specific demethylase 1" (LSD-1) which is an epigenetic regulator of salt-sensitive hypertension. The expression of this gene is only seen in the presence of a higher salt dietary load.

> Our results, from animal studies and two hypertensive cohorts of different ethnicities, support LSD-1's role as an epigenetic mediator of dietary sodium's effect on BP. Interestingly, we did not observe this in the (European American) cohort, despite an identical study protocol ... (this) may suggest a relatively intact dietary salt-LSD-1 relationship and/or compensatory mechanisms operating to dampen penetrance in (European Americans). [6]

Salt sensitivity is defined as significant changes in blood pressure in response to a salt load. Seventy-five percent of all African American patients with hypertension display salt sensitivity compared to 50% across all races with hypertension [7]. The true cause for salt sensitivity in any one patient can be difficult to determine due to a number of comorbid factors that lead to salt sensitivity including obesity, worse renal function, more target organ damage, and lower potassium intake, all of which occur more frequently in African Americans [8]. The combination of these genetic and lifestyle factors gives us the disproportionally high salt sensitivity incidence in African Americans that we see.

There is good evidence that even in the absence of hypertension, elevated dietary sodium can adversely affect multiple target organs and tissues, including the vasculature, kidneys, heart, and brain. For example, increased sodium in patients without hypertension reduced endothelial function while sodium restriction improved endothelial function. Having adequate endothelial flexibility is critical to preventing adverse cardiovascular events as well as end-organ damage [9, 10]. Increased sodium also leads to increased left ventricular wall thickness (and mass) independent of a patient's hypertension status [11, 12]. Sodium restriction has been shown to decrease protein excretion (thus improving kidney function) and blood pressure in African Americans with hypertension [13]. Finally, there is evidence that chronically elevated dietary sodium affects the brain by way of boosting the sympathetic outflow system which increases blood pressure variability and can negatively impact end organs [14, 15].

In all, if you have an African American predominant population, the vast majority of your patients with hypertension are salt sensitive and need counseling related to specific lifestyle modifications they should make. Additionally, salt sensitivity increases with age and is associated with increased mortality independent of a patient's hypertension status [6]. With this in mind, all of your patients need salt restriction counseling.

The good news is that a modest reduction in salt intake (half normal consumption: 5–6 g) for a month has been shown to make significant and sustained reductions in blood pressure [16]. In fact, African Americans showed the most pronounced blood pressure reductions in response to salt restriction with a drop of 8 mm Hg systolic over 4 mm Hg diastolic averaged across as array of studies. These treatment outcomes in African American patients have long supported a propensity for better responses to salt restrictions. When your African American patient is hesitant to start a medication to bring down their mildly elevated blood pressure, spend some time determining how much salt is in their diet, and then explain the great impact a one-half reduction in salt can have. With these nuances in mind, suggesting a decrease in salt in any African American's diet is sound and beneficial advice.

Hypertension control is central to primary, secondary, and tertiary interventions aimed at reducing African American mortality and morbidity from hypertension-related complications. Hypertension occurs earlier in African Americans, is more severe, and more likely to be resistant to therapy [17]. The prevalence of hypertension is 45% in African American males and 46% in African American females compared to 34% and 32% for European Americans males and females, respectively. African Americans are also more likely to have "non-dipping blood pressure" (blood pressure than does not decrease by >10% from daytime to nighttime) and nighttime hypertension on ambulatory blood pressure monitoring [3].

It is also interesting to note that hypertension prevalence was higher among US-born African Americans than among either foreign-born non-Hispanic Blacks or all African-born immigrants of any race or ethnicity. In addition, "being born outside the United States, speaking a language other than English at home, and living fewer years in the United States were each associated with a decreased prevalence of hypertension [3]."

The American College of Cardiology/American Heart Association Task Force on Clinical Practice Guidelines issued a major reset in hypertension management in 2017 by lowering the systolic and diastolic levels for both the diagnosis of hypertension and treatment targets. Data has consistently shown an increase in cardiovascular events with progressively elevated blood pressure.

Observational studies have demonstrated graded associations between higher systolic blood pressure (SBP) and diastolic blood pressure (DBP) and increased CVD risk. In a meta-analysis of 61 prospective studies, the risk of CVD increased in a log-linear fashion from SBP levels <115 mm Hg to >180 mm Hg and from DBP levels <75 mm Hg to >105 mm Hg. In that analysis, 20 mm Hg higher SBP and 10 mm Hg higher DBP were each associated with a doubling in the risk of death from stroke, heart disease, or other vascular disease. [18]

In addition, systematic reviews of hypertension treatment trials, including the findings from the Systolic Blood Pressure Intervention Trial (SPRINT) led by prominent African American researcher and physician, Jackson Wright, Jr., clearly documented the benefit of treating to systolic blood pressure targets well below previously recommended levels in preventing cardiovascular events and all-cause mortality including in African Americans and even in patients over age 75 years of age [19–21]. Thus, a new classification system was proposed which set parameters for blood pressure categories of normal, elevated, stage 1 hypertension and stage 2 hypertension (Fig. 4.1).

This reset of the parameters significantly increases the percentage of African Americans with hypertension to 59% for men and 56% for women, overall [18].

Blood Pressure Category	Systolic Blood Pressure		Diastolic Blood Pressure
Normal	< 120 mm Hg	and	< 80 mm Hg
Elevated	120 -129 mm Hg	and	< 80 mm Hg
Hypertension			
Stage 1	130 - 139 mm Hg	or	80 - 89 mm Hg
Stage 2	$\geq$ 140 mm Hg	or	$\geq$ 90 mmHg

Fig. 4.1 Blood pressure categories (By author)

Being more aggressive with blood pressure control in African Americans makes sense from a number of perspectives given the poor outcomes data for stroke, heart attack, congestive heart failure, and more [22, 23].

When it comes to pharmacotherapy, there are a number of important differences in the African American population that significantly alter your approach to blood pressure control. Evidence from multiple trials suggests that African Americans respond well to thiazide diuretics and calcium channel blockers, and they should be used early and often in hypertensive African Americans [24, 25]. Thiazide-type diuretics (chlorthalidone in this study) were better at reducing blood pressure and preventing cardiovascular events than an ACE inhibitor (lisinopril), or an alpha-adrenergic blocker (doxazosin) in African Americans as found in the "Antihypertensive and Lipid-Lowering Treatment to Prevent Heart Attack" (ALLHAT) trial [17].

For ideal blood pressure control, the thiazide-type diuretic dose should be equivalent to chlorthalidone 12.5–25 mg/day or hydrochlorothiazide 25–50 mg/day because lower doses have not been found to be as effective [17]. Overall, calcium channel blockers (amlodipine) and thiazide diuretics are best in African Americans.

Angiotensin-converting enzyme (ACE) inhibitors and angiotensin II receptor blocker (ARB) medications are less effective in African Americans for blood pressure control [26]. A large cohort of over 400,000 patients done at the New York University School of Medicine compared outcomes in African Americans and European Americans with three distinct groups:

1. ACE inhibitors vs. calcium channel blockers
2. ACE inhibitors vs. thiazide diuretics
3. ACE inhibitors vs. beta-blockers

Their study showed that ACE inhibitors were associated with poorer control of blood pressure in African Americans and observationally associated with a significant increase in stroke, heart failure, and combined cardiovascular disease when compared with calcium channel blockers or thiazide diuretics. The inferior outcomes with angiotensin-converting enzyme inhibitors were largely similar to that of beta blockers in this population [26].

Because ACE inhibitors are commonly listed as "first-line" medications for blood pressure control in national and international guidelines and recommendations, it should be noted that this principally is based on their response in European American populations. Based on these large African American-inclusive studies and a number of considerations (including cost, comorbid conditions, and disease propensities), most guideline recommendations suggest a diuretic and/or a calcium channel blocker as first-line antihypertensive therapy in African Americans.

These large studies also confirmed that African Americans along with Asian-Pacific Islanders have a greater incidence of ACE-related cough and a higher rate of discontinuation due to cough compared to all other racial groups. African Americans were also more prone to develop ACE-associated angioedema and hyperkalemia [26].

The renal-sparing benefits of the ACE and ARB medications persist when used to slow renal function decline (particularly in hypertensive renal disease), and they should still be used prophylactically in African American patients with diabetes with proteinuria [27, 28].

Beta-blockers have long been shown to be significantly less effective in most African Americans and are now not recommended as first-line therapy (in the absence of coronary heart disease or heart failure or unless combined with a diuretic or calcium channel blocker) for blood pressure control [27].

Beta-blockers regain their widespread clinical significance in African Americans in the treatment of myocardial infarctions and systolic heart failure according to guidelines across all other populations [29].

It is important to note that these nuances in the pharmacologic care of hypertensive African Americans is based on the outcomes of multiple well-designed studies over a number of years and truly represents the "standard of care" for this population. A study by Yazdanshenas and colleagues looked at the prescribing patterns of clinicians seeing older African Americans and found that the "(t)reatment of hypertension appears to be inconsistent with the prevailing treatment guidelines for nearly one-third of the aged African Americans." Most of the mismanaged patients were on beta-blockers and ACE inhibitors as monotherapy for hypertension control [30].

Studies have also confirmed that even less intensive interventions (than pharmacotherapy) have helped high-risk African American patients attain better blood pressure control and medication compliance, including:

- Culturally competent provider
- Team-based patient education including providers and allied health professionals
- Appropriate referrals for health conditions and social needs
- Incremental steps approach [31]

These measures help by improving the understanding of the cardiovascular condition, and as trust-building measures that lead to better medication adherence and office follow-up compliance.

Seeing the same provider has also been found to be positively correlated with successful hypertension control. Hypertensive African Americans are significantly less likely than hypertensive European Americans to consistently see the same provider. Setting up clinical visit protocols that encourage provider continuity will improve a number of critical quality measures including hypertension [31].

4.2   Heart Failure

Despite major breakthroughs in the management of systolic heart failure, hospital admissions, morbidity, and mortality continue to rise, with African Americans being the most affected (Fig. 4.2). Unlike hypertension, the pharmacological approach to systolic heart failure has not been significantly stratified by race, despite the fact that this disease is more predominant in the African American population. As rewarding as the pharmacological breakthroughs of ACE inhibitors, ARBs, beta-blockers, spironolactone, and most recently ARB + NRI (angiotensin receptor blocker in combination with neprilysin inhibitor) in reducing mortality, robust studies on these drugs on targeted racial minority groups are lacking. So far some studies including that of Lanfear et al. "Association of Beta Blocker Exposure with Outcomes in Heart Failure Patients Differs between African American and White Patients" show some differences in response of these drugs between European Americans and African Americans [32]. Within the last 30 years it has been shown that hydralazine and isosorbide dinitrate has a significant mortality benefit. The first Veterans Administration Cooperative Vasodilator—Heart Failure Trial (V-HeFT I) showed a significant mortality benefit of hydralazine-isosorbide dinitrate in comparison to placebo—with a greater response in African Americans [33]. This response was later replicated in studies targeting African Americans alone. The second trial (V-HeFT II), which did a head to head trial of hydralazine and isosorbide dinitrate versus enalapril, showed comparative benefit in mortality, ejection fraction, and oxygen consumption [34]. This can raise the possibility of hydralazine/isosorbide dinitrate as a first-line alternative

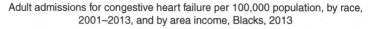

Adult admissions for congestive heart failure per 100,000 population, by race,
2001–2013, and by area income, Blacks, 2013

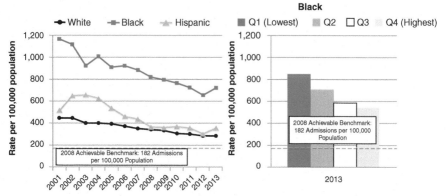

Key: Q1 represents the lowest income quartile and Q4 represents the highest income quartile based on the median income of a patient's ZIP
Code of residence
Source: Agency for Healthcare Research and Quality, Healthcare Cost and Utilization Project, State Inpatient Databases 2001-2013 quality
and disparities analysis files and AHRQ Quality Indicators, modified version 4.4
Denominator: U.S. resident population age 18 and over
Note: For this measure, lower rates are better. White and Black are non-Hispanic. Hispanic includes all races

Fig. 4.2 Adult admissions for congestive heart failure. Chartbook on Health Care for Blacks:
National Healthcare Quality and Disparities Report. https://www.ahrq.gov/research/findings/
nhqrdr/chartbooks/blackhealth/acknow.html

to ACE inhibitors/ARBs in the treatment of heart failure. Currently ACCF/AHA
guidelines dictate the use of hydralazine/isosorbide dinitrite only with the exhaustion
of ACE inhibitors/ARBs and spironolactone in patients with persistent chronic heart
failure (Evidence I, A) or only in African American patients in which ACE inhibitors/
ARBs are intolerable (Evidence IIa, B) [35]. Guidelines however do not address the
possibility of hydralazine/isosorbide dinitrite as a first-line alternative.

Reasons for response differences of vasodilators such as hydralazine/isosorbide
dinitrite in African Americans were postulated to be due to intrinsic responses of
nitric oxide on endothelial function. Research by Cardillo et al. [36] and Stein et al.
[37] showed an attenuated response of nitric oxide-mediated vasodilation in comparison to European Americans—a pathophysiological response that may link to
the increase risk of vascular disease such as hypertension and heart failure. As isosorbide dinitrite and hydralazine affects endothelial nitric oxide metabolism and
degradation, their relationship to race specific endothelial nitric oxide metabolism
has been postulated as a reason for the differential response in African Americans.

One thing to note is that despite the benefit of these vasodilators in African
Americans, the use of these medications in the management of systolic heart failure is suboptimal as seen in the "OPTIMIZE-HF trial" [38]. In comparison to the
other options, these classes are the least promoted in systolic heart failure management and are therefore unlikely to be used. The benefits of the other classes of

drugs in systolic heart failure has been well established, accepted, and practiced for years, while the benefits of vasodilators to many clinicians may still be new. Further emphasis and education on the benefits of this class in systolic heart failure should be encouraged.

In comparison to systolic heart failure where major breakthroughs in pharmacological management have occurred, the progress in the management of heart failure with preserved ejection fraction, previously known as diastolic heart failure, has been much slower. The approach to management—managing the underlying cause while treating symptoms—has been the standard approach. Spironolactone has been the only drug that has shown a mortality benefit in these patients. So far, trials entertaining other drug classes including vasodilators have showed no benefit.

Finally, it should be noted that there are also significant differences in cardiovascular marker laboratory levels between patients of European American and African American backgrounds. The natriuretic peptides, BNP and NT-pro-BNP, are counterregulatory hormones involved in volume homeostasis and cardiovascular remodeling. B-type natriuretic peptide (BNP) levels have been shown to reliably facilitate diagnosis and predict overall prognosis in patients with acute and chronic heart failure. The levels of both markers are predictive of worse cardiovascular disease when elevated. Krim and colleagues found that when hospitalized for heart failure, African Americans and Asian Americans had significantly higher BNP levels [39].

In sharp contrast, the Reasons for Geographic and Racial Differences in Stroke (REGARDS) Study measured the differences in patients *without* significant disease burden and found that African Americans have much lower natriuretic peptide levels. The increased risk for mortality stratification that occurs when BNP and NT-pro-BNP levels increases is still valid across all racial groups, but the baseline level disparities can present potential clinical issues. In short, an elevated BNP and NT-pro-BNP are still positively associated with a worsened prognosis in all races, but African Americans have a significantly lower baseline NT-pro-BNP.

(African American) individuals have a higher prevalence of CV disease; therefore, intuitively they should have higher NTproBNP levels than (European American) individuals, suggesting possible non-hemodynamic mechanisms (eg, decreased production) as a cause for lower NTproBNP levels in (African American) individuals. Taken collectively, the findings of paradoxically low NP levels suggest the likelihood of a primary deficiency among (African American) individuals. [40]

With that deficiency, researchers suggest that lower level natriuretic peptide results in African Americans may convey the wrong assumption regarding cardiac stability in this population. In other words, early heart failure could exist in the presence of "normal-looking" NT-pro-BNP levels.

4.3   Lipids

African Americans have more favorable lipid profiles than matched European Americans including having higher HDL cholesterol levels, lower triglycerides, and lower LDL cholesterol levels, multiple studies have confirmed [41–43]. With disproportionally higher cardiovascular disease in African Americans, researchers have wondered how these better lipid profiles coincide with the documented worse outcomes and is the lipid profile an "under identifier" of African Americans at risk for cardiovascular events. The variability seen based on race and ethnicity is yet another curiosity given clinician's accepted strict association of bad lipids equaling worse outcomes, and good lipids leading to improved outcomes.

> It is clear that there is further complexity in this relationship among African Americans, who have, on average, a more favorable lipid profile compared to European Americans, yet they do not experience an associated decrease in diseases that are expected to be responsive to reduction in this key risk factor. [41]

Years earlier, scientists attributed elevated Lipoprotein Lipase (LPL) levels, the enzyme responsible for hydrolyzing triglycerides, and lower apolipoprotein CIII levels, an atherogenic plaque destabilizer, as principally responsible for the improved cholesterol picture in African Americans. Others have determined that the better lipid profiles in African Americans are not due to diet and lifestyle considerations noting worse fat content in foods consumed and less exercise in African American patient populations compared to European Americans [42].

Attempts to drill down to why good lipids do not lead to better outcomes in African Americans have continued to baffle providers, but the assumption is the impact of other cardiovascular risk factors (hypertension, obesity, and diabetes) overwhelm the beneficial impact of the improved lipid profile.

There are also racial differences in response to diet modifications with African Americans' lipid profiles being less responsive to an unsaturated fat diet than European Americans:

> The controlled study diets lowered plasma apo C-III and triglycerides from concentrations on the participants' usual diets in (European Americans) but not in (African Americans), bringing (European Americans) closer to the low means of (African Americans) and eliminating the large differences between the races in these atherogenic lipoprotein components. We observed that the lack of diet effects on triglycerides and apo C-III in (African Americans) is independent of their lower baseline concentrations. The specific reasons for this cannot be ascertained from this study. Whatever the mechanism, dietary therapies to reduce atherogenic apo C-III and triglyceride that are useful in (European Americans) may not prove to be as successful in (African Americans). However, these diets may still be effective in reducing CHD risk in (African Americans) through reductions in blood pressure, cholesterol, and apo B. [40]

African Americans had lower triglyceride and apolipoprotein CIII levels on their existing diets and were less responsive to diet modifications aimed at lowering these already low plasma levels.

> Although the study diets are useful for reduction of CHD risk by reducing apo B, LDL cholesterol, and blood pressure in both races, they did not lower plasma triglycerides and apo C-III in (African Americans). [43]

Diet modifications do still work in African Americans with salt sensitivity (already discussed) and for LDL cholesterol lowering which can still have a dramatic effect on cardiovascular risk. The overall message is to have a lower threshold for cardio-vascular prophylaxis in spite of a beneficial-looking lipid profile. Any opportunity to lower or eliminate risk factors in African Americans should never be overlooked.

4.4   Atrial Fibrillation

Atrial fibrillation is the most prevalent arrhythmia in the United States and is asso-ciated with significant adverse outcomes that include stroke, heart failure, and increased mortality [44]. Surprisingly, studies also confirm a decreased atrial fibril-lation incidence in African Americans (41% lower risk of being diagnosed than European Americans) but a greatly increased occurrence of stroke and sudden death in African Americans with atrial fibrillation. Some have suggested the decreased incidence is actually under-diagnosis, but others have called it a "racial paradox" where despite atrial fibrillation being a sequelae of increased hypertension, dia-betes, obesity, heart failure, and myocardial infarctions, all of which are higher in African Americans, the incidence of atrial fibrillation is paradoxically lower. African Americans were also less likely to be aware they have atrial fibrillation, and much less likely to be treated with warfarin, and these findings were independent of insurance and socioeconomic class. Significant disparities as it relates to stroke prevention in a stroke-prone population was found in a study by Meschia and col-leagues who looked at over 30,000 patients:

> We also found that among those who were aware that they had AF (atrial fibrillation) and who had confirmation of the diagnosis of AF, (African Americans) were about one quarter as likely to be treated with warfarin as (European Americans). In striking contrast, risk of stroke as stratified by the CHADS$_2$ score was not a predictor of warfarin use. The fact that risk of future stroke did not significantly alter the likelihood of warfarin use would seem to reflect an evidence-practice gap. [45]

The risk for death in the presence of atrial fibrillation in the first 4 months after diag-nosis was very high with CAD, heart failure, and stroke accounting for the majority of deaths, the study also found. Their risk for hospitalization from atrial fibrillation doubled as did the risk for recurrent stroke and related multi-infarct dementia.

4.5   Stroke

As a quarter of all strokes occur in the presence of atrial fibrillation and while representing 13% of the US population [46], African Americans experience almost twice that percentage of all strokes [47]. And when a stroke occurs, African Americans have them earlier in life and present with more severe and disabling conditions [47]. The "Cardiovascular Quality and Outcomes" group concluded that "compared with other race/ethnicity groups, (African American) patients were less likely to receive IV tissue-type plasminogen activator <3 hours, early antithrombotics, antithrombotics at discharge, and lipid-lowering medication prescribed at discharge," a study looking at over 200,000 patients showed [48]. Not surprisingly, with these prescriptive deficiencies in play, data analysis also showed a persistently increased rehospitalization rate in African Americans at both 30 days and 1 year for all causes. African Americans also have a 2.4 times higher rate of recurrent strokes than European Americans in the face of lower secondary prevention measures, and the highest burden of mortality than any racial group [49].

Stroke patients overseen by neurologists were 3.7 times more likely to receive intravenous thrombolysis than those attended to by non-neurologists for all races and ethnicities (study from the Baylor College of Medicine), but unfortunately African Americans were half as likely as European Americans to be seen by a neurologist when presenting with a stroke [49].

Prophylactic aspirin use is also decreased among African Americans as compared to Whites and the indications for aspirin use are actually higher in African Americans. Aspirin reduces the risk of stroke, coronary heart disease, and colorectal cancer at low doses and the risk for gastrointestinal bleed is much lower than the impact of the prevented event. Recommending aspirin use appropriately in African Americans is imperative given the increased incidence of colon cancer, CAD, and strokes in this high-risk, high-event population.

Overall, the US Preventive Services Task Force (USPSTF) recommends referring adults who have cardiovascular disease risk factors and are obese to intense behavioral counseling interventions to promote a healthful diet and physical activity [50]. The CDC reports that 44% of African American men and 48% of African American women have some form of cardiovascular disease thus making almost half of your African American patient population eligible for lifestyle modification counseling [51]. Most insurances pride themselves on covering USPSTF preventative recommendations so there should be no barriers to referring your African American patients to these proven lifestyle modification counselors.

4.6 Peripheral Vascular Disease

Issues relating to racial and ethnic disparities in the treatment, management, and outcomes for patients with peripheral vascular disease and limb ischemia have been well documented [52]. Compared to European American patients, several studies have found that African Americans with peripheral vascular disease are more likely to have amputations of limbs and less likely to have their lower limb correctively revascularized either surgically or via an endovascular approach [52–54]. In another study, African Americans were estimated to be at a 77% higher risk of lower extremity amputation versus revascularization when compared to European American patients [53]. Researchers looked at the differences in treatment of patients and found that European Americans patients sought treatment in the earlier stages of their peripheral vascular disease than African Americans. They added that having more advanced disease at the time of hospital admission, evidenced by a planned outpatient admission versus an emergency department admission, was associated with worse outcomes. African Americans tended toward more emergency department admissions and outpatient generated admissions [55]. The presumption was that the lack of provider access in minorities drove the majority of the difference.

A study of the African Americans in the Jackson Heart Study determined that cigarette smoking was directly linked to peripheral vascular disease, and the correlation of severity was directly linked to the number of cigarettes smoked per day [56]. Moreover, the study determined that African Americans who smoke were at twice the risk for peripheral artery disease that matched European American controls.

> Among current smokers, there was a dose-dependent response whereby those smoking ≥20 cigarettes per day and higher pack-year smoking exposure demonstrated considerably higher odds of subclinical PAD compared with those smoking 1–19 cigarettes per day. [56]

The negative effects of smoking also showed a dose-dependent association with abdominal aorta and aorto-iliac calcification that could lead to obstruction or aneurysmal formation.

4.7   Deep Vein Thrombosis and Pulmonary Embolism

Venous thromboembolism consisting of deep vein thrombosis (DVT) and pulmonary embolism (PE) appear to have a slightly higher incidence in African American patients compared to European Americans [57]. As the third leading cause of vascular death behind myocardial infarction and stroke, venous thromboembolism represents a serious threat to clinical outcomes in the African American community. African Americans have the highest incidence of both provoked (caused by an identifiable risk factor) and unprovoked venous thromboembolism and have the highest short-term mortality. To complicate the situation further, African Americans also have higher major bleeding events when treated for DVT and PE [57].

It has been hypothesized that African Americans have a pro-thrombotic state that may increase susceptibility to DVT and PE due to higher serum concentrations of von Willebrand Factor and Factor VIII [57]. There are distinct differences in anticoagulation with African Americans requiring higher warfarin dosing and having more difficulty staying within a therapeutic range. Currently, there are no adjustments in therapy or duration of anticoagulation after thromboembolism specific to African Americans, but this is mainly due to the lack of research containing a significant number of African Americans to study. Like other disparities in care, racial differences in anticoagulation exist as well.

> (European Americans) generally are more likely to receive anticoagulation than (African Americans) and other racial and ethnic minorities. A retrospective study of a heart failure database showed that (African Americans) were less likely to receive anticoagulation compared to (European Americans) after adjustment for multiple variables including age, sex, history of AF, liver disease, and alcohol use. Analysis of in-hospital mortality among approximately 400,000 patients showed that (African Americans) were less likely to be treated with anticoagulants for AF (OR 0.84; 95% CI: 0.75–0.94). In a population-based study, the odds of (African Americans) being treated with warfarin were only one-fourth as great as (European Americans) (OR 0.28; 95% CI: 0.13–0.60). The racial differences in anticoagulation practice are unexplained and a profound demonstration of racial disparities. [44]

The key is to be vigilant with recommendations for anticoagulation in all indicated disorders, know that African Americans may well be pro-thrombotic, be prepared to use higher doses of warfarin, and err on the side of anticoagulation when in doubt.

Of the contributors to health disparities in cardiovascular care "referral-sensitive procedures such as percutaneous transluminal coronary angioplasty (PTCA) and coronary artery bypass graft (CABG) surgery were amongst those that showed the

Important Differences in Cardiovascular Care

- Studies suggest that obesity and low potassium diet contribute to the higher prevalence of salt sensitivity and show this characteristic can be reversed with weight loss and greater potassium intake.
- Salt sensitivity has been linked to blunted nocturnal blood pressure dipping, decreased endothelial function, proteinuria, and target end-organ damage in African Americans.
- Hypertension therapy should be initiated with a thiazide-type diuretic or a calcium channel blocker which have been proven to have better blood pressure reduction and are better at preventing cardiovascular events.
- ACE inhibitors are less effective at reducing blood pressure and should not be used as monotherapy unless the patient has diabetes with proteinuria.
- Hydralazine and isosorbide dinitrate have proven mortality benefit in African Americans with heart failure with reduced ejection fraction.
- Elevated BNP and NT-pro-BNP are positively associated with a worsened prognosis in all races, but African Americans have a significantly lower baseline NT-pro-BNP.
- African Americans have more favorable lipid profiles but with disproportionately higher cardiovascular disease. Because of this, clinicians should have a lower threshold for cardiovascular prophylaxis.
- African Americans have a greatly increased risk for stroke and recurrent stroke.
- African Americans have a decreased risk for atrial fibrillation and because of the increased risk for stroke, this is referred to as a "racial paradox."
- Recommending low dose aspirin use is imperative given the high incidence of CAD, strokes and colorectal carcinoma.
- Clinicians should be aware that African Americans have an increase susceptibility to venous thromboembolism (and pulmonary embolism) and they should err on the side of using anticoagulation.

greatest disparities" [58]. In other words, providers are widening a number of differences between minority and majority care. While the lack of access to medical insurance or high quality medical technology does drive a number of poor outcomes in cardiovascular care, we providers, through our actions and inactions, drive too many of them. These important and life-saving differences should be embedded in every practice caring for African Americans.

References

1. 2015 National Healthcare Quality and Disparities Report Chartbook on Health Care for Blacks. Rockville: Agency for Healthcare Research and Quality; 2016. AHRQ Pub. No 16-0015-1-EF.
2. Carnethon M, Pu J, Aalbert M, et al. Cardiovascular health in African Americans: a scientific statement from the American Heart Association. Circulation. 2017;136:e393–423.
3. Cooper R, Wolf-Maier K, et al. An international comparative study of blood pressure in populations of European vs. African descent. BMC Med. 2005;3:2.
4. Benjamin E, Blaha M, Chiuve S, et al. Heart disease and stroke statistics-2017 update: a report from the American Heart Association. Circulation. 2017;135(10):e146–603.
5. Young D, Fischer H, Arterburn D, et al. Associations of overweight/obesity and socioeconomic status with hypertension prevalence across racial and ethnic groups. J Clin Hypertens (Greenwich). 2018;20(3):532–40.
6. Williams J, Chamarthi B, Goodarzi M, et al. Lysine-specific demethylase 1: an epigenetic regulator of salt-sensitive hypertension. Am J Hypertens. 2012;25(7):812–7.
7. Richardson S, Freedman B, Ellison D, et al. Salt sensitivity: a review with a focus on non-Hispanic blacks and Hispanics. J Am Soc Hypertens. 2013;7(2):170–9.
8. Wright J, Rahman M, et al. Determinants of salt sensitivity in black and white normotensive and hypertensive women. Hypertension. 2003;42:1087–92.
9. Gates P, Tanaka H, Hiatt W, et al. Dietary sodium restriction rapidly improves large elastic artery compliance in older adults with systolic hypertension. Hypertension. 2004;44:35–41.
10. Todd A, Macginley R, Schollum J, et al. Dietary salt loading impairs arterial vascular reactivity. Am J Clin Nutr. 2010;91:557–64.
11. Jin Y, Kuznetsova T, Maillard M, et al. Independent relations of left ventricular structure with the 24-hour urinary excretion of sodium and aldosterone. Hypertension. 2009;54:489–95.
12. Rodriguez CJ, Bibbins-Domingo K, Jin Z, et al. Association of sodium and potassium intake with left ventricular mass: coronary artery risk development in young adults. Hypertension. 2011;58:410–6.
13. Swift PA, Markandu ND, Sagnella GA, et al. Modest salt reduction reduces blood pressure and urine protein excretion in black hypertensives: a randomized control trial. Hypertension. 2005;46:308–12.
14. Stocker SD, Monahan KD, Browning KN. Neurogenic and sympatho-excitatory actions of NaCl in hypertension. Curr Hypertens Rep. 2013;15:538–46.
15. Parati G, Ochoa JE, Lombardi C, et al. Assessment and management of blood-pressure variability. Nat Rev Cardiol. 2013;10:143–55.
16. He F, Li J, Macgregor G. Effect of longer term modest salt reduction on blood pressure: cochrane systematic review and meta-analysis of randomized trials. BMJ. 2013;346:f1325.
17. Wright J, Probstfield JJ, Cushman W, et al. ALLHAT findings revisited in the context of subsequent analyses, other trials, and meta-analyses. Arch Intern Med. 2009;169(9):832–42.
18. Whelton PK, Carey RM, Aronow WS, et al. 2017 ACC/AHA/AAPA/ABC/ACPM/AGS/APhA/ASH/ASPC/NMA/PCNA guideline for the prevention, detection, evaluation, and management of high blood pressure in adults. J Am Coll Cardiol. 2018;71(6):1269–324.
19. Wright J, Williams J, Whelton P, SPRINT Research Group, et al. A randomized trial of intensive versus standard blood pressure control. N Engl J Med. 2015;373(22):2103–16.
20. Williamson J, Supiano M, Applegate W, et al. Intensive vs standard blood pressure control and cardiovascular disease outcomes in adults aged ≥75 years: a randomized clinical trial. JAMA. 2016;315:2673–82.

21. Still C, Rodriguez C, Wright J, et al. Clinical outcomes by race and ethnicity in the systolic blood pressure intervention trial (SPRINT): a randomized clinical trial. Am J Hypertens. 2017;31(1):97–107.

22. Muacevic A, Adler J, Asad A, et al. American Heart Association high blood pressure protocol 2017: a literature review. Cureus. 2018;10(8):e3230.

23. Wright J, Dunn J, Cutler J, et al. Outcomes in hypertensive black and nonblack patients treated with chlorthalidone, amlodipine, and lisinopril. JAMA. 2005;293(13):1595–608.

24. Materson B, Reda D, Cushman W, et al. Single-drug therapy for hypertension in men – a comparison of six antihypertensive agents with placebo. N Engl J Med. 1993;328:914–21.

25. Trunbull F. Effects of different blood-pressure-lowering regimens on major cardiovascular events: results of prospectively-designed overviews of randomized trials. Lancet. 2003;362(9395):1527–35.

26. Bangalore S, Ogedegbe G, Gyamfi J, et al. Outcomes with angiotensin-converting enzyme inhibitors vs other antihypertensive agents in hypertensive blacks. Am J Med. 2015;128(11):1195–203.

27. National Clinical Guideline Centre. Hypertension: the clinical management of primary hypertension in adults: update of clincal guidlines 18 and 34. London: Royal College of Physicians (UK) - National Clinical Guideline Centre; 2011.

28. Williams S, Nicholas S, Vaziri N, Norris K. African Americans, hypertension and the renin angiotensin system. World J Cardiol. 2014;6(9):878–89.

29. Rizos C, Elisaf M. Antihypertensive drug therapy in patients with African ancestry. Expert Opin Pharmacother. 2014;15(8):1061–4.

30. Yazdanshenas H, Bazargan M, Orum G, et al. Original reports: cardiovascular disease and risk factors. prescribing patterns in the treatment of hypertension among underserved African American elderly. Ethn Dis. 2014;24(4):431–7.

31. Scisney-Matlock M, Bosworth H, Giger J, et al. Strategies for implementing and sustaining therapeutic lifestyle changes as part of hypertension management in African Americans. Postgrad Med. 2009;121(3):147–59.

32. Lanfear D, Hrobowski T, Peterson E, et al. Association of beta blocker exposure with outcomes in heart failure patients differs between African American and white patients. Circ Heart Fail. 2012;5(2):202–8.

33. Cohn J, Archibald D, Francis G, et al. Veterans administration cooperative study on vasodilator therapy of heart failure: influence of prerandomization variables on the reduction of mortality by treatment with hydralazine and isosorbide dinitrate. Circulation. 1987;75(5 Pt 2):IV49–54.

34. Cohn J, Johnson G, Ziesche S, et al. A comparison of enalapril with hydralazine-isosorbide dinitrate in the treatment of chronic congestive heart failure. N Engl J Med. 1991;325:303–10.

35. Yancy C, Jessup M, Bozkurt B, et al. ACC/AHA/HFSA focused update of the 2013 ACCF/AHA guideline for the management of heart failure. Circulation. 2017;136:e137–61.

36. Cardillo C, Kilcoyne C, Cannon R, et al. Racial differences in nitric oxide-mediated vasodilator response to mental stress in the forearm circulation. Hypertension. 1998;31:1235–9.

37. Stein C, Lang C, Nelson R, Brown M, Wood A. Vasodilation in black Americans: attenuated nitric oxide-mediated responses. Clin Pharmacol Ther. 1997;62(4):436–43.

38. Yancy C, Abraham W, Albert N, et al. Quality of care of and outcomes for African Americans hospitalized with heart failure: findings form the OPTIMIZE-HF registry. J Am Coll Cardiol. 2008;51(17):1675–84.

39. Krim S, Vivo R, Krim N, et al. Racial/ethnic differences in B-type natriuretic peptide levels and their association with care and outcomes among patients hospitalized with heart failure: findings from get with the guidelines–heart failure. JACC Heart Fail. 2013;1(4):345–52.

40. Bajaj N, Gutierrez O, Arora G, et al. Racial differences in plasma levels of N-terminal pro-B-type natriuretic peptide and outcomes: the reasons for geographic and racial differences in stroke (REGARDS) study. JAMA Cardiol. 2018;3(1):11–7.
41. Bentley A, Rotimi C. Inter-ethnic variation in lipid profiles: implications for under-identification of African Americans at risk for metabolic disorders. Expert Rev Endocrinol Metab. 2012;7(6):659–67.
42. Pan Y, Pratt C. Metabolic syndrome and its association with diet and physical activity in US adolescents. J Am Diet Assoc. 2008;108(2):276–86.
43. Furtado J, Campos H, Summer A, Appel L, Cary V, Sacks F. Dietary interventions that lower lipoproteins cantaining apolipoprotein C-III are more effective in whites than in blacks: results of the OmniHeart trial. Am J Clin Nutr. 2010;92(4):714–22.
44. Amponash M, Benjamin E, Magnani J. Atrial fibrillation and race – a contemporary review. Curr Cardiovasc Risk Rep. 2013;7(5):336. https://doi.org/10.1007/s12170-013-0327-8.
45. Meschia J, Soliman M, Soliman E, et al. Racial disparities in awareness and treatment of atrial fibrillation: the reasons for geographic and racial differences in stroke (REGARDS) study. Stroke. 2010;41(4):581–7.
46. Marini C, De Santis F, Sacco S, et al. Contribution of atrial fibrillation to incidence and outcome of ischemic stroke. Stroke. 2005;36:1115–9.
47. Roger V, Go A, Lloyd-Jones D, et al. Heart disease and stroke statistics – 2012 update. Circulation. 2012;125(1):e2–e220.
48. Qian F, Fonarow G, Smith E, et al. Racial and ethnic differences in outcomes in older patients with acute ischemic stroke. Circ Cardiovasc Qual Outcomes. 2013;6(3):284–92.
49. Chiou-Tan F, Keng M, Graves D, Chan K, Rintala D. Racial/ethnic differences in FIM scores and length of stay for underinsured patients undergoing stroke inpatient rehabilitation. Am J Phys Med Rehabil. 2006;85(5):415–23.
50. U.S. Preventive Services Task Force. https://www.uspreventiveservicestaskforce.org/Page/Name/uspstf-a-and-b-recommendations/.
51. African American Health. Vital signs. Centers for Disease Control and Prevention. 2017. Accessed 9 May 2019.
52. Bell E, Lutsey P, Basu S, et al. Lifetime risk of venous thromboembolism in two cohort studies. Am J Med. 2016;129(3):339.e19–26.
53. Rowe VL, Weaver FA, Lane JS, Etzioni DA. Racial and ethnic differences in patterns of treatment for acute peripheral arterial disease in the United States, 1998–2006. J Vasc Surg. 2010;51:21S–6S.
54. Durazzo TS, Frencher S, Gusberg R. Influence of race on the management of lower extremity ischemia: revascularization vs amputation. JAMA Surg. 2013;148:617–23. https://doi.org/10.1001/jamasurg.2013.1436.
55. Mustapha J, Fisher B, Rizzo J, et al. Explaining racial disparities in amputation rates for the treatment of peripheral artery disease (PAD) using decomposition methods. J Racial Ethn Health Disparities. 2017;4(5):784–95.
56. Clark D, Cain L, Blaha M, et al. Cigarette smoking and subclinical peripheral arterial disease in blacks of the Jackson heart study. J Am Heart Assoc. 2019;8:e010674.
57. Payne A, Miller C, Hooper W, Lally C, Austin H. High factor VIII, von Willebrand factor, and fibrinogen levels and risk of venous thromboembolism in blacks and whites. Ethn Dis. 2014;24(2):169–74.
58. Bolorunduro O, Kiladejo A, Animashaun I, Akinboboye O. Disparities in revascularization after ST elevation myocardial infarction (STEMI) before and after the 2002 IOM report. J Natl Med Assoc. 2016;108(2):119–23.

Important Differences in the Care of Diabetes and Obesity

5

5.1 Obesity

Disparities in obesity and diabetes foreshadow important differences in health outcomes including long-term disability, cardiovascular disease, some cancers, and premature mortality. African Americans have a significantly increased rate of obesity even starting in the school-age populations and before [1, 2]:

> Between the ages of 2 and 5 years, the proportion of (African American) children with a body mass index (BMI) at or above the 95th percentile is 11.3%, twice the proportion for (European American) children, and these differences persist through development (3.5%). Such findings suggest obesity-related risk factors present during early childhood may give rise to the differences observed through development. [3]

The widespread prevalence of obesity is best represented by the following map of the United States showing almost nationwide obesity rates higher than 35% in the vast majority of states (Fig. 5.1).

Because the increased obesity rate leads to elevated diabetes diagnosis, we find that African Americans have an across-the-board increased rate of diabetes as compared to European Americans for all education levels. From the much earlier diagnosis of type 2 diabetes in younger African Americans to the increased occurrence of diabetes-induced heart failure and other related hospitalizations, the burden of obesity in African Americans is heavy and starts very early in life [3].

One of the most impactful risk factors for obesity is having obese parents. Children with obese parents are ten times more likely to be obese. Through example, obese parents pass on unhealthy eating habits like increased intake of sugary beverages, higher fast food consumption, and diets that contain higher starch-content foods. Obese parents also have a more sedentary lifestyle with

© Springer Nature Switzerland AG 2020
G. L. Hall, *Patient-Centered Clinical Care for African Americans*,
https://doi.org/10.1007/978-3-030-26418-5_5

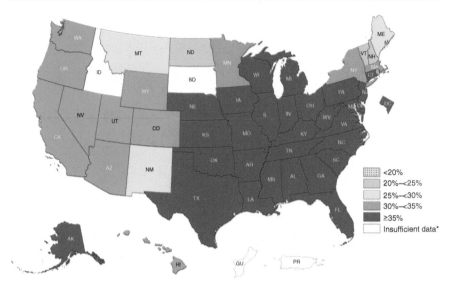

Fig. 5.1 Prevalence of self-reported obesity among African Americans adults by state and territory, BRFSS, 2016–2018. https://www.cdc.gov/obesity/data/prevalence-maps.html

significantly less exercise and more watching television than their European American counterparts. Because early childhood is a critical period for habit-forming and body fat distribution formation, these environment influences have lifelong consequences [4].

In general, African American women have a higher prevalence of obesity and are at a greater risk for weight management problems [5]. This increased propensity for obesity is directly correlated with increased chronic illnesses. Providers struggle with approaches to obese African American women given social norms that may encourage some degree of higher weight acceptance. Studies have consistently found self-size satisfaction occurs at a higher weight among African Americans than matched European Americans. While 74% of African Americans have a BMI greater than 25, compared to 67% of European Americans, the percentage that are unhappy with their weight is significantly lower [5]. Patients seeking bariatric consultation show a disproportionally lower number of African Americans "interested" in surgery. Even weight loss after bariatric surgery is more modest for African Americans due to the more tempered weight-loss goals [6]. Christina Wee and colleagues at the Beth Israel Deaconess Medical Center looked at obese patients considering bariatric surgery:

men were less likely than women and African Americans were less likely than (European American) primary care patients to have seriously considered bariatric surgery after accounting for sociodemographic factors and comorbid conditions. Much of the observed differences by race, however, appeared to be explained by higher QOL (quality of life) scores among African American relative to (European American) patients with obesity. [6]

This increased quality of life shows the greater acceptance of some degree of obesity in African Americans and is reflected in their more conservative targets for ideal body weight. Multiple studies show that African Americans have a higher "ideal" body weight than other races, and this increased comfort at a higher weight drives down their desire for dramatic weight loss [6]. These attenuated goals for weight loss are reflected even after bariatric surgery such that there are conflicting reports as to whether bariatric surgery is less effective in African Americans [7] with a number of studies showing a comparatively less overall weight loss [8]. Although weight loss is greater in European Americans, significant weight loss still occurs in African Americans having gastric bypass surgery. If your patient would benefit from bariatric surgery, studies have shown that having the primary care provider suggest the procedure rather than waiting for patient self-directed referrals has shown increased success.

As a disproportional number of African Americans live in higher violence neighborhoods, there has been growing evidence of a link between increased stress from growing up in violent areas and subsequent obesity [9]. A study by Assari and others at the University of Michigan found a direct link between increased adolescent fear of violence and subsequent obesity in adulthood.

Fear of violence in the neighborhood at age 15 is predictive of an increase in BMI from age 21 to 32 among female but not male African American youth. Thus for female African American youth who live in disadvantaged areas, fear of violence in the neighborhood is one of the contributing factors of their increased risk of obesity. [9]

It has long been accepted that psychogenic stress can lead to excess body fat and obesity, although the exact mechanism has remained elusive. Some suggest cortisol as a mediator and others put forth other hypotheses [10].

Be aware that the increased obesity we see in inner city African American women (and men) is not completely self-induced, and approaching the patient with an accusatory tone and simple instructions to "lose weight" ignores the laundry list of contributing causes with some of them starting before birth.

5.2   Diabetes Type 2

Diabetes occurs at a disproportional rate in African Americans and they are 80% more likely to be diagnosed than European Americans, and the occurrence is slightly higher in women [11]. Of those with diabetes, there is a higher propensity for related end-organ damage than European Americans. The prevalence of visual impairment, end-stage renal disease, wound-related leg amputations, and overall hospitalizations are dramatically higher in African Americans with diabetes [11]. The CDC reports that African American men die at over twice the rate of any other race gender group from hyperglycemic crises [12].

Hospital admissions for uncontrolled diabetes is dramatically higher for African Americans across all income groups [13]. Diabetes is diagnosed at an earlier age (median age 49 vs. 55.4 in European Americans), and this earlier age is significant because the development of diabetes complications is directly related to both glycemic control and overall duration of disease (Fig. 5.2).

Diabetes remains the most common cause of kidney failure across all races and is an important contributory factor with African Americans. Kidney disease is already more prevalent in African Americans due to hypertension-related causes [12].

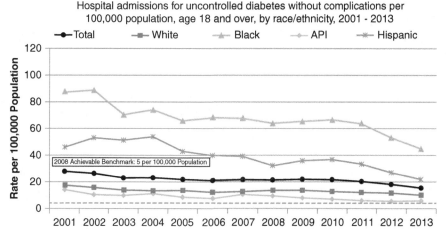

Key: API = Asian or Pacific Islander
Source: Agency for Healthcare Research and Quality, Healthcare Cost and Utilization Project, State Inpatient Databases, 2001– 2013 quality and disparities analysis files and AHRQ Quality indicators, modified version 4.4.
Denominator: U.S. resident population age 18 and over.
Note: For this measure, lower rates are better. Rates are adjusted by age and gender using the total U.S. resident population for 2010 as the standard population; when reporting is by age, the adjustments is by gender only.

Fig. 5.2 Hospital admissions for uncontrolled diabetes by race/ethnicity. Chartbook on Health Care for Blacks: National Healthcare Quality and Disparities Report. https://www.ahrq.gov/research/findings/nhqrdr/chartbooks/blackhealth/acknow.html

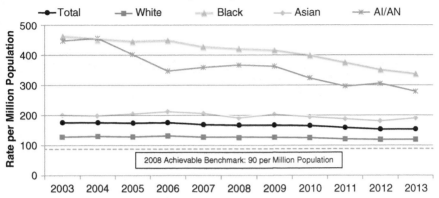

New cases of end-stage renal disease due to diabetes, per million population, by ethnicity, 2003-2013

Fig. 5.3 New cases of end-stage renal disease due to diabetes by race/ethnicity. Chartbook on Health Care for Blacks: National Healthcare Quality and Disparities Report. https://www.ahrq.gov/research/findings/nhqrdr/chartbooks/blackhealth/acknow.html

Keeping blood sugars in the normal range and using renal-protective medications (ACE and ARB) in patients with diabetes has been shown to slow the occurrence and progression of renal disease. Just in a 10-year span, significant progress has been made in decreasing new cases of renal disease, but unfortunately significant disparities persist (Fig. 5.3).

Most research pertaining to African Americans and diabetes points to increased insulin resistance and upregulated beta cell function when compared to European Americans. To some extent, African Americans are more prone to develop diabetes genetically, but external factors like obesity, poor diet, and smoking contribute much more.

5.2.1 Smoking

A large study consisting of over 5000 African Americans found that those African Americans who smoke more than a pack of cigarettes in a day were at increased risk for diabetes [14]. The study group included current heavy smokers, former smokers, and "never" smokers, all of whom were African Americans, and followed them over the course of several visits. At the end of the study, they looked to see who had developed diabetes. Both former and nonsmokers had similar occurrences, which is good news for people who have stopped smoking. Those participants who smoked more than a pack a day of cigarettes had a much higher occurrence of developing diabetes (up to 40% higher). The increased smoking was associated with "impaired pancreatic beta cell function." The researchers go on to say:

> Although smoking cessation should be encouraged for everyone, certain high-risk groups such as (African Americans) who are disproportionately affected by diabetes mellitus should be targeted for cessation strategies. [14]

There is fairly consistent evidence that smoking leads to increased diabetes in other racial populations as well including the "Nurses' Health Study" [15] and the "Insulin Resistance Atherosclerosis Study" [16]. Both of these large studies showed substantial increased diabetes in current smokers. Given that one in five African Americans smoke and the rate of diabetes is higher for other reasons, adding diabetes as a deterrent or motivation to stop smoking can be very impactful.

5.2.2 HbA1c Differences

HbA1c at diagnosis is generally a point higher in African Americans (8.9 in European Americans and 9.8 in African Americans), and when controlling for socioeconomic status, quality of care, self-management behaviors, and access, African Americans still have higher HbA1c levels [17]. A study by Saaddine et al. looked at NHANES data for participants' age 5–24 years and found that African American youths consistently had higher HbA1c levels [18]. Another researcher found the same persistently high HbA1c levels even "after controlling for age, sex, BMI, maternal BMI, and poverty-income ratio" [19].

In all, HbA1c value differences in African Americans essentially equates to a 0.4% difference (higher) for glucose matched European American patients. A HbA1c of 7.5% should be interpreted as 7.1% in African Americans and a HbA1c of 6.5% should raise concerns for a higher risk of hypoglycemia, particularly in the elderly. This difference across a population could change the threshold for diabetes diagnosis and for targeted control in African Americans. Thus the accepted relationship between HbA1c and the "mean blood glucose" used by clinicians and laboratories is different for African Americans:

> The relationship between mean blood glucose and HbA1c may not be the same in all people. Indeed, the published regression line from the "A1c-Derived Average Glucose" (ADAG) Study demonstrated a wide range of average glucose levels for individuals with the same HbA1c levels. [17]

Given the additional "wiggle-room" implicit in the across-the-board elevations in HbA1c levels in African Americans, some have suggested a wider "rule-in and rule-out" range in African Americans with levels lower than 5.5% representing the absence of diabetes and levels higher than 7% clearly confirming the diagnosis. Levels within the "wiggle-room" should be further investigated with glucose plasma testing or glucose tolerance measurements. Because of the limitations of HbA1c measurements in some clinical pictures (uremia and hemolytic anemia for example) and the racial differences discussed above, some of the patients with a HbA1c level between 5.5% and 7% will clearly have diabetes, and others will not [20]. To assume that those African Americans in that range are now "borderline" and to withhold treatment would also be a great mistake. The simple fact is the HbA1c is less accurate and dependable at "near-normal" levels and any result in this range should prompt additional confirmatory studies [19].

Another curiosity with HbA1c has to do with patients with sickle cell trait:

Among African Americans from 2 large, well-established cohorts, participants with SCT (sickle cell trait) had lower levels of HbA_{1c} at any given concentration of fasting or 2-hour glucose compared with participants without SCT. These findings suggest that HbA_{1c} may systematically underestimate past glycemia in (African American) patients with SCT and may require further evaluation. [21]

Given that one in ten African Americans have sickle cell trait, it is important to consider their trait when interpreting the results of a HbA1c and if your suspicions warrant, consider additional glucose tolerance testing before making broad assumptions based on the HbA1c outcome.

Once diabetes has been confirmed, studies show about a third to half of your African American patients will be non-adherent with whatever treatment you prescribe [22, 23]. Adherence to prescribed medications varies according to a number of confounding and compounding variables including access, trust for provider, medication cost, health literacy, psychological barriers, insulin preconceptions, and regime complexity.

A study of focus groups of African Americans found a high degree of skepticism regarding their own diabetes diagnosis *"as if somehow ... a mistake in diagnosis had been made"* [24]. Taking the time to explain how the diabetes diagnosis was made incorporating their presenting symptoms with an explanation of what the elevated glucose does to the body over time should help proactively convince the certainty of the diagnosis. That same focus group study found a significant number of the participants felt personally responsible for their diabetes and that "responsibility" was out of proportion to factors actually in their control. Many participants felt that if they could have adequately controlled their diet, they never would have gotten the disease … and if they could control their diet going forward, the diabetes would go away.

Fatalism in African Americans with diabetes is common, and this attitude of hopelessness as it relates to diabetes control is "significantly associated with poor medication adherence and self-care" as found by Walker and colleagues at the Medical University of South Carolina [25].

> After adjustment for pertinent covariates, the relationship remained statistically significant for the association between increased diabetes fatalism, decreased medication adherence, and decreased levels of three self-care behaviors (diet, exercise, and blood sugar testing). [25]

Clarifying the misconceptions regarding the patient's ability to control their diabetes without medications will allow the patient to progress beyond this barrier to accepting medications as a viable option to care. While diet, exercise, and proper medications are central to diabetes care, they are not mutually exclusive in most African American patients, or anyone else for that matter. Diabetes education with every new patient with diabetes is essential to dispelling false impressions and preconceptions regarding the cause and ultimate control of the disease.

Studies have repeatedly shown that increased diabetes knowledge and understanding have been positively associated with better glycemic control and increased education leads to elevated confidence in the patient's ability to achieve control [26]. This increased confidence, also referred to as "self-efficacy," has also been associated with better "glycemic control, medication adherence, self-care, and mental health-related quality of life". Demystifying diabetes through education individually and in small groups has been shown to improve overall diabetes care [25].

> Health care providers are urged to explore the person's knowledge about the diagnosis, ask about past experiences with others who have diabetes, and inquire as to their feelings and beliefs about the purpose of prescribed medication and dispel any myths. [24]

5.3   Diabetes Type 1

The incidence of type 1 diabetes in African Americans is lower than in European descent Americans, but those with early onset type 1 diabetes mellitus are at high risk for severe diabetic nephropathy and end-stage renal disease. While type 1 diabetes typically develops from autoimmune destruction of pancreatic beta cells, there is a subset of African American individuals who are phenotypically type 1 (thin and insulin-dependent) but do not have the immunologic markers indicative of an autoimmune destruction process. These patients have insulin deficiency but not from an immune process, and their diabetes is ketosis-prone. This non-immune type 1 diabetes is more prevalent in African Americans.

5.4   Diabetes Medication Adjustments

Unlike the significant differences in African American's response to hypertension medications, there is little evidence to suggest a similar landscape in diabetes medications. What researchers have found is a propensity among clinicians to be slow when advancing or intensifying diabetic therapy. Having a *clinician care flow sheet* that anticipates the progression of medications typically used to achieve control will remove mental barriers clinicians may subconsciously erect that prevents the acceleration of care. Sometimes providers "stall" adding additional medications (or increasing a dose). This *slow-to-prescribe* behavior is sometimes referred to as "clinical inertia" and mimics the added energy needed to set an object in motion. By knowing what medication or next dose choice well in advance of its need, clinicians will simplify their thought process and expedite ultimate glycemic control.

5.5   Diet Management Approaches

Type 2 diabetes is a complicated disease with variable presentations and idiosyncratic causes that vary from patient to patient. As their clinician, we have the unique opportunity to personalize the explanation of their diabetes diagnosis and tailor the approach to care in a very specific manner. Obtaining a diet history from the patient with analysis of calories from foods and beverages with specific stepwise recommendations will allow for a graduated, and better tolerated, change [27]. If, for example, your patient drinks a 2 liter bottle of their favorite soda on a daily basis (not an unusual example), they consume almost 1000 calories through that source alone. Cutting 1000 calories from anyone's diet is a major accomplishment and certainly a significant step in the right direction. Many African American patients will appreciate sequential and specific recommendations that target easily identifiable foods, and only represent a slight change in their overall diet (at first). For our example, an easy, impactful, and significant initial diet modification could be:

• Stop all sugary beverages.

This clear instruction would impact dietary calories, be relatively easy to accomplish, and provide a positive outcome in glycemic control. It will not achieve full control of the diabetes but will be a great first step.

It has also been clearly proven that telling patients *what not to eat* leads to more confusion of what is allowable and worse outcomes with compliance [27]. Dariush Mozaffarian looked at dietary trends and priorities for patients at risk for, or already diagnosed with, diabetes, obesity, and cardiovascular diseases. Quite simply, he affirmed what nutritionists are now emphasizing:

> evidence-informed dietary priorities include increased fruits, non-starchy vegetables, nuts, legumes, fish, vegetable oils, yogurt, and minimally processed whole grains; and fewer red meats, processed (e.g., sodium-preserved) meats, and foods rich in refined grains, starch, added sugars, salt, and trans fat. [28]

Nutrition recommendations are also moving away for banning specific foods and moving toward looking at the combinations of foods in a diet that work synergistically toward better health. And better emphasizing healthy patterns in a diet versus its calorie composition:

> These lines of evidence indicate that an "energy imbalance" concept of obesity is oversimplified. Whereas short-term weight loss can be achieved by any type of calorie-reduced diet, in the long-term, counting calories may not be biologically nor behaviorally relevant. Rather, the quality and types of foods consumed influence diverse pathways related to weight homeostasis, such as satiety, hunger, brain reward, glucose-insulin responses, hepatic *de novo* lipogenesis, adipocyte function, metabolic expenditure, and the microbiome. Thus, all calories are not equal for long-term adiposity: certain foods impair pathways of weight homeostasis, others have relatively neutral effects, and others promote the integrity of weight regulation. [28]

By giving one or two specific dietary category instructions per visit, adjustments in the overall diet seem less radical to the patient and more easy to follow. At a subsequent office visit, and after success with curtailing the soda pop consumption, suggestions for increasing fruit or nut consumption can be initiated. This is framed with the patient's preferences in fruit (or nuts) elucidated, and then eliciting their agreement to the plan. It is critical to get the patient's endorsement of the diet recommendation during the visit. Simply telling the patient to start eating an orange every day, and then leaving the exam room defeats the purpose. Getting a diet history of likes and dislikes, aligning their diet plan with proven recommendations, and then gradually moving their habits to better alignment, is the best approach to sustained diet modification. The clinician will also need to stress that follow-up recommendations will be forthcoming regarding other aspects of their diet, but for now, the prime directive is whatever they have indicated, and be as helpful with specifics as needed.

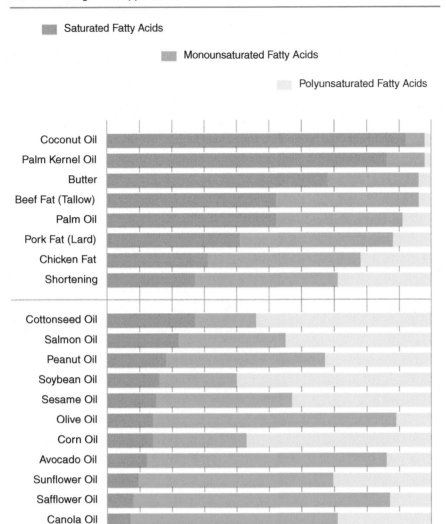

Fig. 5.4 Comparison of fats and oils. The Dietary Guidelines for Americans 2015–2020. National Diabetes Education Program. https://health.gov/dietaryguidelines/2015/guidelines/chapter-1/a-closer-look-inside-healthy-eating-patterns/#callout-dietaryfats

For example, when preparing meals, a modest change in the quality of oils used for food preparation can have a great impact on the overall health content of a meal (Fig. 5.4). With the goal to decrease the saturated fats in a diet, talk about the different compositions of oils, their experiences with them and some practical applications with food they already eat.

5.6   Marketing Competition

Products associated with significant population-wide morbidity in diabetes (sodas, candy, and alcoholic beverages) are advertised disproportionately in magazines, billboards, and television advertisements targeting African Americans when compared with any other racial audience [29]. Advertisements for "healthier food and beverage products" (fruits, vegetables, low-fat meats, soy, and dairy products) are disproportionately underrepresented in African American communities [28–31].

Trying to have an impact on the dietary wants of a patient with that kind of marketing barrage is like trying to explain to your children that an amusement park is not as fun as the television commercials make it seem. The important take-home message is … your message(s) will need reinforcement and repetition, and the trust of the conveyor of the message will absolutely impact its acceptance.

Important Differences in the Care of Diabetes and Obesity
- African Americans have a significantly increased rate of obesity which directly correlates to an increased risk for chronic illnesses.
- African American women have a higher prevalence of obesity and are at a greater risk for weight management problems.
- African American children with obese parents are ten times more likely to be obese.
- African Americans are more than 80% likely to be diagnosed with diabetes type 2 than European Americans and are also diagnosed at an earlier age.
- Ensuring optimal blood sugar control as well as utilizing renal protective medications have been shown to slow the progression of renal disease.
- HbA1c value differences in African Americans essentially equates to a 0.4% difference (higher) for glucose matched European American patients.
- HbA1c is less accurate and dependable at "near-normal" levels in African Americans.
- Patients with sickle cell trait have lower HbA_{1c} at any given level.
- HbA1c is not reliable in patients with sickle cell disease or thalassemia.
- African Americans should be encouraged to stop smoking as smoking increases the risk of diabetes in this population.
- Adequate diabetes education both in small groups and individually has been shown to improve overall diabetes care.
- Advising patients on food and beverage use using a stepwise recommendation will allow for a graduated, better tolerated and accepted change.

References

1. Guerrero A, Mao C, Fuller B, Bridges M, Franke T, Kuo A. Racial and ethnic disciplines in early childhood obesity: growth trajectories in body mass index. J Racial Ethn Health Disparities. 2016;3(1):129–37.

2. Abraham P, Kazman J, Zeno S, Deuster P. Obesity and African Americans: physiologic and behavioral pathways. ISRN Obes. 2013;2013:314295.

3. Fuemmeler B, Stroo M, Lee C, Bazemore S, Blocker B, Ostbye T. Racial differences in obesity-related risk factors between 2-year-old children born of overweight mothers. J Pediatr Psychol. 2015;40(7):649–56.

4. Taveras E, Gillman M, Kleinman K, Rich-Edwards J, Rifas-Shinman S. Racial/ethnic differences in early life risk factors for childhood obesity. Pediatrics. 2010;125(4):686. https://doi.org/10.1542/peds.2009-2100.

5. Bruce M, Sims M, Miller S, Elliott V, Ladipo M. One size fits all? Race, gender and body mass index among US Adults. J Natl Med Assoc. 2007;99(10):1152–8.

6. Wee C, Davis R, Jones D, et al. Sex, race, and the quality of life factors most important to patients' well-being among those seeking bariatric surgery. Obes Surg. 2016;26(6):1308–16.

7. Anderson W, Greene G, Forse R, Apovian C, Istfan N. Weight loss and health outcomes in African Americans and whites after gastric bypass surgery. Obesity (Silver Spring). 2007;15(6):1455–63.

8. Buffington C, Marema R. Ethnic differences in obesity and surgical weight loss between African Americans and Caucasian females. Obes Surg. 2006;16(2):159–65.

9. Assari S, Lankarani M, Caldwell C, Zimmerman M. Fear of neighborhood violence during adolescence predicts development of obesity a decade later: gender differences among African Americans. Arch Trauma Res. 2016;5(2):e31475.

10. Bjorntorp P. Do stress reactions cause abdominal obesity and comorbidities? Obes Rev. 2001;2(2):73–86.

11. U.S. Department of Health and Human Services Office of Minority Health. Diabetes and African Americans. https://minorityhealth.hhs.gov/omh/browse.aspx?lvl=4&lvlid=18.

12. Becles G, Chou C. Diabetes – United States, 2006 and 2010. MMWR Morb Mortal Wkly Rep. 2013;62(03):99–104.

13. Chartbook on Health Care for Blacks. Agency for Healthcare Research and Quality, Rockville. https://www.ahrq.gov/research/findings/nhqrdr/chartbooks/blackhealth/acknow.html.

14. White W, Cain L, Benjamin E, et al. High-intensity cigarette smoking is associated with incident diabetes mellitus in black adults: the Jackson Heart Study. J Am Heart Assoc. 2018;7(2):Pii: e007413.

15. Zhang L, Curhan G, Hu F, Rimm E, Forman J. Association between passive and active Smoking and incident type 2 diabetes in women. Diabetes Care. 2011;34(4):892–7.

16. Foy C, Bell R, Farmer D, Goff D, Wagenknecht L. Smoking and incidence of diabetes among US adults. Diabetes Care. 2005;28(10):2501–7.

17. Herman W, Cohen R. Racial and ethnic differences in the relationship between HbA1c and blood glucose: implications for the diagnosis of diabetes. J Clin Metab. 2012;97(4):1067–72.

18. Saaddine J, Fagot-Campagna A, Rolka D, et al. Distribution of HbA1c levels for children and young adults in the U.S.: third National Health and nutrition examination survey. Diabetes Care. 2002;25(8):1326–30.
19. Eldeirawi K, Lipton R. Predictors of hemoglobin A1c in a national sample of nondiabetic children: the third National Health and nutrition examination survey, 1988–1994. Am J Epidemiol. 2003;157(7):624–32.
20. Ziemer D, Kolm P, Weintraub W, et al. Glucose-independent, black-white differences in hemoglobin A1c levels: a cross-sectional analysis of 2 studies. Ann Intern Med. 2010;152(12):770–7.
21. Lacy M, Wellenius G, Sumner A, et al. Association of sickle cell trait with hemoglobin A1c in African Americans. JAMA. 2017;217(5):507–15.
22. Shenolikar R, Balkrishnan R, Camacho F, Whitmire J, Anderson R. Race and medication adherence in medicaid enrollees with type 2 diabetes. J Natl Med Assoc. 2006;98(7):1071–7.
23. Kyanko K, Franklin R, Angell S. Adherence to chronic disease medications among New York City medicaid participants. J Urban Health. 2013;90(2):323–8.
24. Bockwoldt D, Staffileno B, Coke L, et al. Understanding experiences of diabetes medications among African Americans living with type 2 diabetes. J Transcult Nurs. 2017;28(4):363–71.
25. Walker R, Smalls B, Hernandez-Tejada M, Campbell J, Davis K, Egede L. Effect of diabetes fatalism on medicaition adherence and self-care behaviors in adults with diabetes. Gen Hosp Psychiatry. 2012;34(6):598–603.
26. Bains S, Egede L. Associations between health literacy, diabetes knowledge, self-care behaviors, and glycemic control in a low income population with type 2 diabetes. Diabetes Technol Ther. 2011;13(3):335–41.
27. The Dietary Guidelines for Americans 2015–2020. National Diabetes Education Program. https://www.cdc.gov/diabetes/ndep/pdfs/dietary_guidelines_slides.pdf. Accessed 9 May 2019.
28. Mozaffarian D. Dietary and policy priorities for cardiovascular disease, diabetes, and obesity. A comprehensive review. Circulation. 2016;133:187–225.
29. Yancey A, Cole B, Brown R, et al. A cross-sectional prevalence study of ethnically targeted and general audience outdoor obesity-related advertising. Milbank Q. 2009;87(1):155–84.
30. Outley CW, Taddese A. A content analysis of health and physical activity messages marketed to African American children during after-school television programming. Arch Pediatr Adolesc Med. 2006;160(4):432–5.
31. Tirodkar MA, Jain A. Food messages on African American television shows. Am J Public Health. 2003;93(3):439–41.

Important Differences in Cancer Care

6

African Americans have the highest mortality for the top five causes of cancer death [1]. Figure 6.1 shows African Americas edge out European Americans in lung cancer and pancreatic cancer but substantially outnumber deaths in colon, breast, and most significantly prostate cancer. The reasons for these and other cancer disparities are not simple nor easily explained, but a better understanding of current hypotheses and best practices may improve your patient's outcomes.

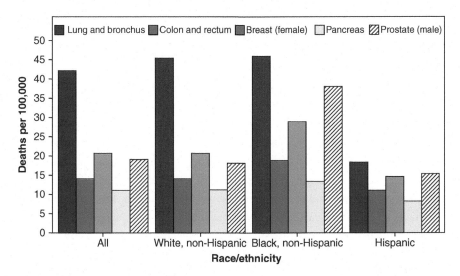

Fig. 6.1 Mortality rate for top five cancers by Race/Hispanic Ethnicity. QuickStats: age-adjusted death rates for top five causes of cancer death, by Race/Hispanic Ethnicity—United States, 2014 [1]

© Springer Nature Switzerland AG 2020
G. L. Hall, *Patient-Centered Clinical Care for African Americans*,
https://doi.org/10.1007/978-3-030-26418-5_6

6.1   Breast Cancer

The incidence of breast cancer is higher among European American women at 129 per 100,000, while the African American rate is slightly lower at 125 per 100,000. The breast cancer mortality for African American women is 30 deaths per 100,000 women, while European American women have 21 deaths per 100,000 women. Nationally, African American women were 43% more likely to die from breast cancer than their European American counterparts, yet the disease occurs less [2, 3].

A study of almost 20,000 cancer patients of the Southwest Oncology Statistical Center found results that "when controlled for uniform stage, treatment, and follow up, African American sex-specific cancers (breast, ovarian, and prostate) still did worse" [4]. The startling nature of this outcome might initially suggest that clinicians are powerless to have an impact on these cancers, but in reality, more vigorous surveillance and research, coupled with more aggressive therapy, is the simple answer. For breast cancer, most studies verify that increased mammography, chemotherapy, and hormone therapy (if indicated) will lead to decreased mortality.

In all, African Americans tend to have breast cancer tumors with worse prognostic factors including higher stage and lower frequency of hormone receptor-positive tumors that are more easily treated with medications available [5]. African American women have more estrogen- and progesterone-negative tumors and thus suffer a twofold lower survival compared with tumors having both receptors as positive. Even among those African Americans with estrogen receptor-positive tumors, the rate of recurrence was twice that of European Americans.

There is almost uniform consensus that obesity adds to all-cause mortality in patients with breast cancer, and given the increased obesity in African American women, the worsened outcomes in this population may, at least partially, be explained by this. Add the increased mortality and morbidity in breast cancer to the long list of reasons for weight loss in your obese African American patients.

Among African American women, increased knowledge of the benefits of early detection can and do lead to improved outcomes. In addition, false perceptions of the diagnosis of cancer can negatively impact outcomes and decrease engagement. A study from Drew University of Medicine and Science looked at perceptions about cancer and early detection in African American women.

> Given that 5-year survival rates range from 84% to 93% for all three cancers (breast, cervical, and colorectal) if detected early, our data suggest that a substantial proportion of African American women in South Los Angeles are not aware of the benefits of early detection, particularly for colorectal and cervical cancers. For these two types of cancers, almost one out of two African American women in our study believed that chances of survival are fair or poor, even if the cancer was detected early. Our findings confirm results from

previous studies that have identified fatalistic attitudes towards cancer outcomes among African American women and the attitude that cancer is a death sentence [6].

Patient education involving the specifics of why a screening test is done and what advantage is gleaned is essential when ordering a test. Frequently, African Americans are not aware of the true value of finding a cancer early versus just "finding a cancer." Many have the (perfectly understandable) perspective that they "do not want to find a cancer in them" and the benefit of finding the cancer early is lost on many because of the fatalistic misconceptions they hold. Explain the benefit and what is avoided by having a mammogram, Pap test, or colonoscopy early and the dramatic differences in survival from finding a localized cancer versus one that has spread. These conversations, although time consuming, can also be life-saving.

6.2   Colon Cancer

African American men and women continue to have higher colorectal cancer incidence and mortality rates and are diagnosed at more advanced stages than European Americans. Even when adjustments are made for socioeconomic status, African Americans still have significantly lower screening [7]. The colon cancer incidence and death rate is so high in the African American community that the American College of Gastroenterology recommends screening begin at age 45 rather than the age 50 recommendation for the rest of the US population [8]. This recommendation was confirmed by Paquette et al. who did a retrospective database review of all patients with colon cancer from 2000 through 2011, and given the cancer stage at discovery, he concluded that African Americans would benefit significantly from earlier surveillance [9]. The lower screening rate in African Americans has also been postulated as a cause for finding more advanced cancers upon diagnosis, but researchers are also looking into other causes for these more aggressive cancers. Studies also showed an increased occurrence in African Americans for right-sided colon cancer tumors prompting recommendations against sigmoidoscopy in these patients because a significant number of tumors would be missed [10]. That recommendation, which was ratified by the American College of Gastroenterology, was issued in 2005:

> The committee recommends colonoscopy as a "first line" screening procedure for colorectal cancer for African Americans rather than the flexible sigmoidoscopy because of the high overall risk and as well as some evidence that African Americans have more right-sided cancers and polyps. March 21, 2005 American College of Gastroenterology. [8]

Because most colorectal cancers progressed from colorectal adenomas, screening can potentially impact a great number of patients. As primary providers shift their attention from treatment to prevention, the potential impact financially, in terms of lives saved, and suffering prevented, becomes palpable.

Another large study looking at over 60,000 Medicare recipients found that interval colorectal cancer after a screening colonoscopy was more common in African American patients and it occurred more frequently with gastroenterologists with high polyp detection rates [11]. The assumption is providers with lower polyp detection rates could have missed precancerous lesions at the original colonoscopy and are the reason for some of these new cancers being found. Another contributing factor is faster-growing interval cancers that aggressively grew in between procedures and presumably needed sooner surveillance than occurred. The study also suggested that screening parameters may need to be adjusted based on race in order to minimize the added cancer risk.

Spending the time to properly convince a patient of the potential benefit of preventive measures is critical, and with colon cancer screening, the options have widened to much less invasive procedures.

With fecal DNA testing, colonoscopy, CT colonography, and annual fecal immunochemical testing (FIT), there are an array of options from which your patients can choose. Studies have found that having a trained patient navigator (tailored navigation) help patients with these options will increase compliance among African Americans significantly [12]. Whereas "tailored navigation" failed to show significant benefit in predominant European American populations, it has fairly consistently been seen as a benefit in African American populations [13]. In addition, leaving the options freely open for the patients to choose (colonoscopy, CT colonography, or FIT DNA, etc.) versus strongly stressing one particular option improved compliance and follow-through with African Americans.

Computer-delivered tailored interventions with African Americans have also been reviewed in a number of studies, and most have shown a significant positive impact in changed perception of colorectal screening or actual screening behavior [14, 15]. As discussed later in the book, presentations that are delivered in the form of stories connect better, are easier to remember, and tend to more positively impact behavior. With more use of electronic medical records, having a computer screen in the exam room on which to present an educational video is becoming less of a barrier. Tailoring the video, as much as possible, to the specifics of the patients' history also helps ultimate success. Showing a video tailored to African Americans and discussing screening options and outcomes provide another objective source of useful information that the patient can add to your thoughtful advice.

6.3   Prostate Cancer

Financially, finding an aggressive cancer later in stage is costlier to society than finding it earlier. Advanced cancers put a serious strain on our medical system and our ability to distribute limited healthcare dollars. So what is the sense in screening these high-risk, high cost diseases less? A commonly held perception is that prostate cancer is an indolent disease and most that get it die from other unrelated causes. While this may be the case across multiple populations, prostate cancer occurs earlier, is more aggressive, and ultimately kills African American men at a much higher rate.

In a stunning move, the United States Preventive Services Task Force (USPSTF) issued guidelines recommending that all male patients, irrespective of race, no longer be routinely screened for prostate cancer with a prostate-specific antigen (PSA) test [16]. An amended guideline issued in May 2018 suggests that men age 55–69 engage in an individualized decision-making process with their physician.

> For men aged 55 to 69 years, the decision to undergo periodic prostate-specific antigen (PSA)–based screening for prostate cancer should be an individual one. Before deciding whether to be screened, men should have an opportunity to discuss the potential benefits and harms of screening with their clinician and to incorporate their values and preferences in the decision. Screening offers a small potential benefit of reducing the chance of death from prostate cancer in some men. However, many men will experience potential harms of screening, including false-positive results that require additional testing and possible prostate biopsy; over diagnosis and overtreatment; and treatment complications, such as incontinence and erectile dysfunction. In determining whether this service is appropriate in individual cases, patients and clinicians should consider the balance of benefits and harms on the basis of family history, race/ethnicity, comorbid medical conditions, patient values about the benefits and harms of screening and treatment-specific outcomes, and other health needs. Clinicians should not screen men who do not express a preference for screening. [16]

The Task Force goes on to recommend *against* PSA-based screening for prostate cancer in men 70 years and older [16].

A detailed review of the USPSTF guideline research used to draw these conclusions shows that they were based on two studies, one of which reported that only 4% of its participants were African American and the other had no demographic information but used participants from seven European countries with small African American populations [17].

Unfortunately, some insurances have begun not paying for PSA measurements in their enrollees in support of the USPSTF decree and as a way to deter clinicians from ordering the test [18]. Experts in urology that see larger African American populations have questioned these short-sighted guidelines and asked that they be revised as soon as possible [19].

In response, the USPSTF issued additional advice regarding the PSA and African Americans.

Based on the available evidence, the USPSTF is not able to make a separate, specific recommendation on PSA-based screening for prostate cancer in African American men. Although it is possible that screening may offer greater benefits for African American men compared with the general population, currently no direct evidence demonstrates whether this is true. Screening, and subsequent diagnosis and treatment, has the potential to increase exposure to potential harms. Decision analysis models suggest that given the higher rates of aggressive prostate cancer in African American men, PSA-based screening may provide greater benefit to African American men than the general population. These models also suggest a potential mortality benefit for African American men when beginning screening before age 55 years. The USPSTF believes that a reasonable approach for clinicians is to inform African American men about their increased risk of developing and dying of prostate cancer as well as the potential benefits and harms of screening so they can make an informed, personal decision about whether to be screened. Although the USPSTF found inadequate evidence about how benefits may differ for African American men, it recognizes the epidemiologic data showing that African American men may develop prostate cancer at younger ages than average-risk men and understands that some African American men and their clinicians will continue to screen at younger ages. The USPSTF does not recommend screening for prostate cancer in men, including African American men, older than 70 years. [20]

Unfortunately, this parenthetical advice is not easily accessed on the USPSTF website, but it clearly represents a more nuanced modification in the recommendations.

The course of prostate cancer has been shown to be different in African American men, prostate cancer volume is greater in African American men, and advanced metastatic prostate cancer occurs at a stunning 4:1 ratio when compared to European American men. The more aggressive nature of prostate cancer in African American men has prompted some to think the cancer has an augmented growth rate. Because of this increased growth rate, African American men present at a later stage of disease than age-matched European American patients. African American men also have higher PSA values and higher PSA density when compared to European Americans, and some have suggested this is linked to a higher tumor burden [19].

The American Urological Association has listed African American race as a risk factor for prostate cancer:

The Panel recognizes that certain subgroups of men age 40 to 54 years may realize added benefit from earlier screening. For example, men at increased risk for prostate cancer, such as those with a strong family history or those of African-American race, may benefit from earlier detection, given their higher incidence of disease. [17]

Statements such as these are found within urologic guideline summaries that essentially advise against widespread PSA screening, but if your patient population is African American, an entirely different screening approach is "assumed" due to your knowledge of the prostate cancer difference in African Americans.

By not acknowledging that different populations require different approaches in America, well-meaning initiatives may actually cause more suffering. The overarching message in most urological guidelines is to decrease PSA screening, and the parenthetical exception is … but not in African Americans and people with strong family histories. Unfortunately, these parenthetical exceptions are frequently lost to most readers, and the overarching message (stop PSA measurements) is reported in media and summary statements for wide distribution.

Prostate cancer in African American men is the most prevalent occurring cancer and the second most common cause of overall cancer deaths. When compared to European Americans, we see an entirely different prevalence and mortality rates. The prostate cancer incidence is 70% higher in African American men. Similarly, the mortality from prostate cancer is 2.4 times higher than European American men. Given that there is no cure for metastatic prostate cancer, finding it sooner in populations at risk for early metastasis is the only logical course.

Screen for prostate cancer early and regularly in the African American male population.

6.4 Lung Cancer

While the rate of lung cancer in African Americans looks comparable to European Americans at first glance with African American and European American men having an identical 1 in 13 probability of diagnosis (and European woman having higher incidence of 1 in 15 versus 1 in 19 for African American women), the age-adjusted lung cancer incidence is 32% higher in African Americans [21]. Fundamentally, lung cancer is diagnosed 3 years earlier in African Americans [22]. In addition, African Americans are diagnosed more often with lung cancer in intermittent and light smokers when compared to European Americans despite the fact that on average they start smoking later in life.

While smoking is the main driver of lung cancer, there are other causes including alcohol consumption, decreasing BMI, radon exposure, geography, and more. Interestingly, a Kaiser Permanente Medical Care Cohort found that while drinking three glasses of alcohol a day was associated with an increased risk for lung cancer in European Americans, it was not associated with increased risk in African Americans [23]. Living near industrial sources of pollution is associated with increased lung cancer mortality, and African Americans disproportionately fit this demographic. Additionally, industrial exposure is associated with even higher rates of lung cancer in African Americans than would be predicted, essentially showing the same potentiated effect tobacco exposure has in the otherwise less-exposed African American population [24, 25].

In terms of lung cancer subtypes, non-small cell cancers still compose the majority of lung cancers in African Americans, but there is a 30% increased risk for adenocarcinoma and a 70% increased squamous cell carcinoma within that category. Overall the incidence of small cell carcinoma tends to be lower in African Americans [24].

With the acceptance of low-dose computed tomography (LDCT) as a reimbursed annual screening for the early detection of lung cancer in adults 55–80 years with a 30-pack-year history (and currently smoke or have quit within the last 15 years), we can expect a significant reduction in lung cancer mortality overall simply due to early detection [26]. But with African Americans starting smoking later in life, smoking fewer cigarettes, having more advanced tumors at diagnosis, and living more in industry-dense locations, many with substantially increased lung cancer risk will more likely be deemed screening ineligible. Katki and colleagues at the National Institutes of Health have proposed using a risk-based model that considers demographics and other risk factors that could potentially avert any widening of disparities unintentionally produced by broad recommendations [26].

6.5   Equitable Tobacco Cessation Advice

Studies have shown that smoking cessation improves when providers discuss the topic at clinical encounters [27, 28]. That discussion, and its focus and intensity, varies across providers. Only half (48%) of African American smokers reported receiving advice to quit from physician providers (2010 National Health Interview Survey), and the rate for advising European Americans was better, but not by much (52%) [29]. With the widespread health impact and societal cost of tobacco use and abuse, advising only half of smokers to stop smoking is a missed clinical opportunity of monumental proportions. Julia Soulakova found African Americans are twice as likely to profess an intention to quit smoking after getting advice to quit than European Americans [30]. Another study by Kulak and others found distinct racial differences in smoking cessation with African Americans having more attempts to quit and European Americans being significantly more successful in quitting [31]. Making the time to discuss the merits of quitting and reviewing the various strategies available for African Americans takes full synergistic advantage of their increased motivation to attempt to quit.

6.5.1   African American Smoking Paradox

Among African Americans, there is a curious and deadly paradox that has confounded researchers. Alexander and colleagues comment:

> Despite their social disadvantage, African American youth have lower smoking prevalence rates, initiate smoking at older ages, and during adulthood, smoking rates are comparable to (European Americans). Smoking frequency and intensity among African American youth and adults are lower compared to (European Americans) and American Indian and Alaska Natives, but tobacco-caused morbidity and mortality rates are disproportionately higher. Disease prediction models have not explained disease causal pathways in African Americans. [32]

European American male smokers consume 30–40% more cigarettes than their African American counterparts, but African American male smokers are 34% more likely to develop lung cancer. This higher incidence based on lower exposure highlights the imperative of smoking cessation campaigns. An equitable approach would dictate that clinicians spend a disproportionately high amount of time on smoking cessation in African Americans because preventing the initiation of smoking and promoting complete cessation can have a dynamic impact on a patient population.

Studies have also shown a higher propensity among African Americans to smoke mentholated cigarettes (80%) and a higher risk of stroke in that subpopulation [33]. Smoking cessation, for unknown reasons, among menthol cigarette smokers is worse in both African American and Hispanic/Latino smokers, and for those who stopped, fewer were able to remain abstinent [34, 35]. Studies also suggest that it is easier to start smoking a menthol cigarette and there is a higher rate of progression to an established smoker. Menthol cigarettes are more heavily marketed in younger, poorer, and more African American or Hispanic/Latino communities [36, 37].

With 80% of deaths from lung cancer deemed smoking-related, and half of all deaths from cancers of the mouth, esophagus, and urinary bladder caused by smoking, and worse cessation rates among African Americans, a deliberate clinical plan needs to be organized to better educate African Americans that smoke. A start in the discussion is to assess what baseline knowledge exists related to lung cancer and the other risks. Studies have shown that "low income and limited education adversely affect cessation attempts and that often (African American) smokers underestimate the link between cancer and tobacco smoking compared with (European American) smokers" [23]. Successful smoking cessation processes include:

- Clinician-led discussions
- Pertinent educational videos for the patient to see while waiting for their visit
- Patient navigator educational support and discussions

On average, male smokers die 13 years earlier than male nonsmokers, and female smokers die 14 years earlier than female nonsmokers. Saving those years represents an indelible impact on someone's life. What else in medicine can we effect so significantly?

6.6   Multiple Myeloma

Multiple myeloma (MM), a neoplasm of plasma cells, is the most common hematologic malignancy in African Americans with two to three times the incidence of European Americans. The overall incidence rates of multiple myeloma increase with age, particularly after age 40, and are higher in men, particularly African American men. Family history, radiation exposure, workplace exposure, and Agent Orange exposure all place an increased risk for multiple myeloma [38]. A National Cancer Institute study also found that the age of onset of multiple myeloma occurred at significantly younger ages in African Americans [39].

Because of the stark racial differences in the age of onset and the prevalence of multiple myeloma in African American, geneticists began to look for trends and dissimilarities. What they found were specific differences in the genetics of the myeloma cells that varied by race [40]. Overall African Americans had a genetic version of multiple myeloma that occurred more often but also was consistent with better susceptibility to current therapeutic modalities and, therefore, improved outcomes [40]. The increased mortality of multiple myeloma in African Americans is related to the pure increased occurrence, whereas the improved survival is within the entire population with multiple myeloma. More African Americans with multiple myeloma lead to higher mortality, even in the presence of better survival outcomes.

Monoclonal gammopathy of undetermined significance (MGUS) is a precursor to multiple myeloma and is one of the most common premalignant plasma cell disorders. MGUS indicates the presence of a monoclonal immunoglobulin called an M-protein at a level less than 10% clonal bone marrow plasma cells. Greater than 10% of these cells (and associated symptoms) confirms the diagnosis of multiple myeloma. MGUS occurs at a threefold higher rate in African Americans compared to European Americans, but the rate of progression to multiple myeloma is equal [41]. In other words, all racial groups progress from MGUS to multiple myeloma at the same rate, but African Americans have a significantly increased risk to develop MGUS. The racial disparity in the occurrence of MUGUS is present even after adjusting for socioeconomic status [42].

The overall conclusion regarding the "racial disparities" in multiple myeloma rests in a theory best summarized by Greenberg et al.:

> Although MM is clinically considered as a unique disease, it is likely a collection of several cytogenetically unique malignancies that are considered together as one entity solely, because they arise from plasma cells and have roughly similar clinical features. As the racial disparity in the incidence of MM is marked (relative risk of ≥2 in African Americans), it is unlikely that the increase in risk is shared by all cytogenetic subtypes of the disease. Our hypothesis is that the racial predisposition in MM is driven largely by an excess risk of one or more specific cytogenetic subtypes of MM. [41]

The classic clinical manifestations of multiple myeloma include hypercalcemia (>11 mg/dL), renal failure, anemia, and lytic bone lesions as well as greater than 10% clonal bone marrow plasma cells. Patients frequently present with bone pain, pathologic fractures, and recurrent bacterial infections.

After diagnosis, patients are risk stratified and began on chemotherapy and/or bone marrow transplantation. Unfortunately, African Americans are less likely to receive adequate treatment for multiple myeloma including getting newer medications or bone marrow transplants [43–46] Drs. Mark Fiala and Tanya Wildes looked at racial disparities in patient choice and utilization for multiple myeloma and found that African Americans were 37% less likely to choose stem cell transplantation and 21% less likely to utilize bortezomib (a newer more targeted MM medication) than European Americans after controlling for access barriers and overall health status [47]. This difference in patient decision-making as it relates to treatment options impacts cancer outcomes overall.

6.7 "Chemotherapy"

Chemotherapy as a treatment option is a scary word for any patient to hear. Multiple studies have demonstrated significant delays in the initiation and completion of chemotherapy predict inferior outcomes [48–52]. African Americans may have a cultural aversion to the word "chemotherapy" that makes them less likely to agree to this potentially life-saving treatment. Because of a history of seeing their African

American family and friends "get cancer" and then "get chemotherapy" and then lose weight and hair and then die, an unfortunate direct association of chemotherapy with death ensues. The specifics of the cancer and the chemotherapy are frequently lost on many patients.

As providers, it is our responsibility to explain the vast differences in cancers and why and how they occur, as well as clarify that all chemotherapies are not equal nor equivalent in effectiveness or side effects. In fact, all of the medications that a patient takes, from over-the-counter to prescriptions, are a form of "chemotherapy." Encourage the patient to ask questions about their options and ways to minimize adverse reactions. Too many African Americans are saying "no to chemotherapy"

Important Differences in Cancer Care
- Breast cancer incidence is lower in African American women, while the mortality is significantly higher.
- African Americans tend to have breast cancer tumors with worse prognostic factors.
- African Americans have a lower frequency of hormone receptor-positive tumors in breast cancer.
- Increased knowledge of the benefits of early detection of breast cancers lead to improved outcomes among African American women.
- African American women tend to believe their prognosis, when cancer is detected, is much worse than reality.
- The American College of Gastroenterology recommends colorectal screening in African Americans to begin at 45.
- Sigmoidoscopy is contraindicated in African Americans due to a propensity to have more right-sided polyps.
- In African Americans prostate cancer occurs earlier, is more aggressive, and has a higher mortality rate.
- The PSA (prostate-specific antigen) is a more sensitive and specific test for prostate cancer in African Americans.
- African Americans are more likely to smoke menthol cigarettes and therefore inhale more deeply and absorb more nicotine, making it harder to quit.
- African Americans are more likely to develop lung cancer if they smoke; therefore, it is imperative that clinicians spend more time discussing smoking cessation.
- Lung cancer is diagnosed at younger ages, is more advanced, and occurs in lighter smokers in African Americans.

- Living near industrial sources of pollution is associated with increased lung cancer mortality stressing the importance of a more detailed history in regard to geography.
- African Americans have a 30% increased risk for adenocarcinoma and a 70% increase in squamous cell carcinoma of the lung compared to European Americans.
- The US Preventive Services Task Force (USPSTF) recommends annual screening for lung cancer with low-dose computed tomography in adults aged 55–80 years who have a 30-pack-year smoking history and currently smoke or have quit within the past 15 years.
- Multiple myeloma, a neoplasm of plasma cells, is the most common blood-based malignancy in African Americans with two to three times the incidence of European Americans.
- Age of onset of multiple myeloma is significantly younger in African Americans.
- African Americans have a genetic version of multiple myeloma that occurs more often but also is consistent with better susceptibility to current therapeutic modalities and, therefore, improved outcomes.
- MGUS occurs at a threefold higher rate in African Americans compared to European Americans, but the rate of progression to multiple myeloma is equal.
- African Americans may have a cultural aversion to the word "chemotherapy" that makes them less likely to agree to this potentially life-saving treatment in a timely manner.

before getting the information they need. As the cancer progresses, many change their minds, but worse outcomes can now be predicted because of a potentially avoidable delay.

References

1. QuickStats: age-adjusted death rates for top five causes of cancer death, by Race/Hispanic Ethnicity — United States. MMWR Morb Mortal Wkly Rep. 2016;65:989. https://doi.org/10.15585/mmwr.mm6536a10.
2. Centers for Disease Control and Prevention. Breast cancer rates among black and white women. https://www.cdc.gov/cancer/dcpc/research/articles/breast_cancer_rates_women.htm.

 3. American Cancer Society. Breast cancer facts & figures 2017–2018. Atlanta: American Cancer Society, Inc; 2017.
 4. Albain K, Unger J, Crowley J, Coltman C, Hershman D. Racial disparities in cancer survival among randomized clinical trials patients of the southwest oncology group. J Natl Cancer Inst. 2009;101(14):984–92.
 5. Newman L, Stark A, Chitale D, et al. Association between benign breast disease in African American and white American women and subsequent triple-negative breast Cancer. JAMA Oncol. 2017;3(8):1102–6.
 6. Bazargan M, Lucas-Wright A, Jones L, et al. Understanding perceived benefit of early cancer detection: community-partnered research with African American women in South Los Angeles. J Women's Health (Larchmt). 2015;24(9):755–61.
 7. Ananthakrishnan A, Schellhase K, Sparapani R, Laud P, Neuner J. Disparities in colon cancer screening in the Medicare population. Arch Intern Med. 2007;167(3):258–64.
 8. Rex D, Johnson D, Anderson J, et al. Colorectal cancer screening. Am J Gastroenterol. 2009;104:739–50.
 9. Paquette I, Ying J, Shah S, Abbott D, Ho S. African Americans should be screened at an earlier age for colorectal cancer. Gastrointest Endosc. 2015;82(5):878–83.
10. Chattar-Cora D, Onime G, Valentine I, Cudjoe E, Rivera L. Colorectal cancer in a multi-ethnic urban group: its anatomical and age profile. Int Surg. 2000;85(2):137–42.
11. Fedewa S, Flanders W, Ward K, et al. Racial and ethnic disparities in interval colorectal cancer incidence: a population-based cohort study. Ann Intern Med. 2017;166(12):857–66.
12. Myers R, Sifri R, Daskalakis C, et al. Increasing colon cancer screening in primary care among African Americans. J Natl Cancer Inst. 2014;106(12):dju344.
13. Myers R, Bittner-Fagan H, Daskalakis C, et al. A randomized controlled trial of a tailored navigation and a standard intervention in colorectal cancer screening. Cancer Epidemiol Biomark Prev. 2013;22(1):109–17.
14. Rawl S, Skinner C, Perkins S, et al. Computer-delivered tailored intervention improves colon cancer screening knowledge and health beliefs of African Americans. Health Educ Res. 2012;27(5):868–85.
15. Jerant A, Sohler N, Fiscella K, et al. Tailored interactive multimedia computer programs to reduce health disparities: opportunities and challenges. Patient Edu Couns. 2011;85:323–30.
16. U.S. Preventative Services Task Force. Published final recommendations. https://www.uspreventiveservicestaskforce.org/. Accessed 9 May 2019.
17. Shenoy D, Packiananthan S, Chen A, Vijayakumar S. Do African American men need separate prostate cancer screening guidelines? BMC Urol. 2016;16:19.
18. Vastag B. Government task force discourages routine testing for prostate cancer. The Washington Post. https://www.washingtonpost.com/national/health-science/government-task-force-discourages-routine-testing-for-prostate-cancer/2012/05/21/gIQAhFMFgU_story.html?utm_term=.f763e7e5dfb0, 21 May 2012. Accessed 9 May 2019.
19. Carter H, Albertsen P, Barry M, et al. Early detection of prostate cancer: AUA guideline. J Urol. 2013;190(2):419–26.
20. US Preventative Services Task Force, Grossman DC, Curry SJ, et al. Screening for prostate cancer: US Preventative Services Task Force recommendation statement. JAMA. 2018;319(18):1901–13.
21. Lathan C, Waldman BE, Gagne J, Emmons K. Perspectives of African Americans on lung cancer: a qualitative analysis. Oncologist. 2015;20(4):393–9.

22. American Cancer Society. Cancer facts & figures for African Americans 2016–2018. Atlanta: American Cancer Society, Inc; 2016.
23. Ryan B. Lung cancer health disparities. Carcinogenesis. 2018;39(6):741–51.
24. Tran H, et al. Predictors of lung cancer: noteworthy cell type differences. Perm J. 2013;17:23–9.
25. Luo J, et al. Environmental carcinogen releases and lung cancer mortality in rural-urban areas of the United States. J Rural Health. 2011;27:342–9.
26. Katki H, Kovalchik S, Berg C, Cheung L, Chaturvedi A. Development and validation of risk models to select ever-smokers for CT lung cancer screening. JAMA. 2016;315(21):2300–11.
27. Stead L, Buitrago S, Preciado N, et al. Does advice from doctors encourage people who smoke to quit. Cochrane. https://www.cochrane.org/CD000165/TOBACCO_does-advice-from-doctors-encourage-people-who-smoke-to-quit.
28. Dhumal G, Pednekar M, Gupta P, et al. Quit history, intentions to quit, and reasons for considering quitting among tobacco users in India: findings from the wave 1 TCP India survey. Indian J Cancer. 2014;51(01):S39–45.
29. Danesh D, Paskett E, Ferketich A. Disparities in receipt of advice to quit smoking from health care providers: 2010 National Health Interview Survey. Prev Chronic Dis. 2014;11:e131.
30. Soulakova J, Li J, Crockett L. Race/ethnicity and intention to quit cigarette smoking. Prev Med Rep. 2017;5:160–5.
31. Kulak J, Cornelius M, Fong G, Giovino G. Differences in quit attempts and cigarette smoking abstinence between whites and African Americans in the United States: literature review and results from the International Tobacco Control US Survey. Nicotine Tob Res. 2016;18(Suppl 1):S79–87.
32. Alexander L, Trinidad D, Sakuma K, et al. Why we must continue to investigate menthol's role in the African American smoking paradox. Nicotine Tob Res. 2016;18(Suppl 1):S91–101.
33. Gandhi K, Foulds J, Steinberg M, Lu S, Williams J. Lower quit rates among African Americans and Latino menthol cigarette smokers at a tobacco treatment clinic. Int J Clin Pract. 2009;63(3):360–7.
34. Delnevo CD, Gundersen DA, Hrywna M, et al. Smoking-cessation prevalence among U.S. smokers of menthol versus non-menthol cigarettes. Am J Prev Med. 2011;41:357–65.
35. Nonnemaker J, Hersey J, Homsi G, et al. Initiation with menthol cigarettes and youth smoking uptake. Addiction. 2013;108:171–8.
36. Henriksen L, Schleicher NC, Dauphinee AL, et al. Targeted advertising, promotion, and price for menthol cigarettes in California high school neighborhoods. Nicotine Tob Res. 2012;14:116–21.
37. Moreland-Russell S, Harris J, Snider D, et al. Disparities and menthol marketing: additional evidence in support of point of sale policies. Int J Environ Res Public Health. 2013;10:4571–83.
38. Greenberg AJ, Vachon CM, Rajkumar SV. Disparities in the prevalence, pathogenesis and progression of monoclonal gammopathy of undetermined significance and multiple myeloma between blacks and whites. Leukemia. 2012;26(4):609–14.
39. Waxman AJ, Mink PJ, Devesa SS, et al. Racial disparities in incidence and outcome in multiple myeloma: a population-based study. Blood. 2010;116:5501–6. https://doi.org/10.1182/blood-2010-07-298760.
40. Kumar S, Fonseca R, Ketterling RP, et al. Trisomies in multiple myeloma: impact on survival in patients with high-risk cytogenetics. Blood. 2012;119(9):2100–5.

41. Greenberg AJ, Philip S, Paner A, et al. Racial differences in primary cytogenetic abnormalities in multiple myeloma: a multi-center study. Blood Cancer J. 2015;5:e271. https://doi.org/10.1038/bcj.2014.91.
42. Landgren O, Rajkumar SV, Pfeiffer RM, et al. Obesity is associated with an increased risk of monoclonal gammopathy of undetermined significance (MGUS) among African American and Caucasian women. Blood. 2010;116(7):1056–9.
43. Costa LJ, Huang JX, Hari PN. Disparities in utilization of autologous hematopoietic cell transplantation for treatment of multiple myeloma. Biol Blood Marrow Transplant. 2015;21(4):701–706.v.
44. Hari PN, Majhail NS, Zhang MJ, et al. Race and outcomes of autologous hematopoietic cell transplantation for multiple myeloma. Biol Blood Marrow Transplant. 2010;16:395–402.
45. Joshua TV, Rizzo JD, Zhang MJ, et al. Access to hematopoietic stem cell transplantation: effect of race and sex. Cancer. 2010;116:3469–76.
46. Al-Hamadani M, Hashmi SK, Go RS. Use of autologous hematopoietic cell transplantation as initial therapy in multiple myeloma and the impact of socio-geo-demographic factors in the era of novel agents. Am J Hematol. 2014;89:825.
47. Fiala MA, Wildes TM. Racial disparities in treatment use for multiple myeloma. Cancer. 2017;123:1590–6.
48. Biagi JJ, Raphael M, King WD, et al. The effect of delay in time to adjuvant chemotherapy (TTAC) on survival in breast cancer (BC): a systematic review and meta-analysis. ASCO Meet Abstr. 2011;29(15_suppl):1128.
49. Colleoni M, Bonetti M, Coates AS, The International Breast Cancer Study Group, et al. Early start of adjuvant chemotherapy may improve treatment outcome for premenopausal breast cancer patients with tumors not expressing estrogen receptors. J Clin Oncol. 2000;18(3):584–90.
50. Kim YW, Choi EH, Kim BR, et al. The impact of delayed commencement of adjuvant chemotherapy (eight or more weeks) on survival in stage II and III colon cancer: a national population-based cohort study. Oncotarget. 2017;8(45):80061–72.
51. Salazar MC, Rosen JE, Wang Z, et al. Association of delayed adjuvant chemotherapy with survival after lung cancer surgery. JAMA Oncol. 2017;3(5):610–9.
52. Petrelli F, Zaniboni A, Ghidini A, et al. Timing of adjuvant chemotherapy and survival in colorectal, gastric, and pancreatic cancer. A systemic review and meta-analysis. Cancers (Basel). 2019;11(4):Pii: E550. https://doi.org/10.3390/cancers11040550.

Important Differences in Renal Disease

As discussed earlier, renal disease in African Americans is the most dramatically different prevalence of a disorder and results in significant disability, morbidity, and mortality. As end-stage renal disease is principally a result of diabetes and hypertension, and given the increased prevalence of both in African Americans, there is at least a threefold increased occurrence of renal disease in African Americans [1] (Fig. 7.1). Prior to 1994, hypertension was the most common cause of end-stage renal disease in African Americans, but with progressive obesity, diabetes became the leading cause [2, 3]. The excess burden of kidney disease (both diabetic and nondiabetic) has been largely explained by genetic variants in the apolipoprotein 1 (APOL1) gene in African Americans [4, 5]. This increased renal-risk variant emanates from sub-Saharan African ancestors associated with a survival advantage conferred against African sleeping sickness (trypanosomiasis) [3, 4].

The APOL1 genetic variant is found in more than 30% of African Americans and largely absent in European Americans [4]. It is hypothesized that this gene offered protection from *Trypanosoma brucei* carried by the Tsetse fly and was the vector for African sleeping sickness (African trypanosomiasis), an otherwise deadly disease if untreated [4–7]. Through natural selection those with the APOL1 (a functional gene for apolipoprotein L1) had a trypanolytic factor in their serum that conferred natural resistance to the disease. The population with the APOL1 gene was completely immune to African sleeping sickness, while those without the gene lacked protection from the disease. In Africa the APOL1 gene modification was extremely beneficial and provided life-saving protection from a widespread insect-mediated infectious disease that was almost impossible to avoid, but now, in America, it presents a significant long-term renal disadvantage. But once on dialysis, investigators at the Center for Kidney Disease Research and Epidemiology in

© Springer Nature Switzerland AG 2020
G. L. Hall, *Patient-Centered Clinical Care for African Americans*,
https://doi.org/10.1007/978-3-030-26418-5_7

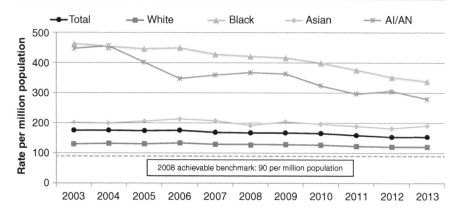

Key: AI/AN = American Indian or Alaska Native
Source: National Institute of Diabetes and Digestive and Kidney Diseases, U.S. Renal Data System, 2003–2013
Denominator: U.S. resident population
Note: For this measure, lower rates are better. Rates are adjusted by age, sex, and interaction of age and sex.
Adjusted rates use the 2011 ESRD cohort as reference

Fig. 7.1   New cases of end-stage renal disease due to diabetes per million population, by ethnicity, 2003–3013. Chartbook on Health Care for Blacks: National Healthcare Quality and Disparities Report. https://www.ahrq.gov/research/findings/nhqrdr/chartbooks/blackhealth/acknow.html

California found that there was a relative survival advantage in African American dialysis patients that was also related to the APOL1 gene variation. The APOL1 gene is associated with increased kidney failure but also associated with better outcomes once on dialysis [8].

With the increased renal disease, African Americans make up 35% of all patients on chronic dialysis [9]. The preferred options for kidney failure are home dialysis or ideally kidney transplantation, but the most common approach is center-based hemodialysis. Center-based hemodialysis involves traveling to a facility three times per week for the nurse-supervised multi-hour procedure. This approach can negatively impact the ability to keep employment as well as lower the overall quality of life. Mehrotra and colleagues looked at racial and ethnic disparities in home dialysis access and use and found that African Americans had a 60% lower rate of home hemodialysis and a 47% lower peritoneal dialysis rate when compared to European Americans [10]. This analysis also demonstrated that African Americans had better mortality rates with these modes of dialysis [10].

Vascular access for hemodialysis also remains inadequate for too many African Americans. Nee and colleagues found that African Americans and Hispanic/Latinos were less likely to initiate hemodialysis with an arteriovenous fistula "independent of predialysis nephrology care, area-level income, dual-eligibility status and other insurance types" [11].

African Americans are less likely to have had a nephrology evaluation prior to kidney failure [11]. An appropriate referral to a specialist can positively impact quality of care.

> The involvement of a nephrologist throughout the more advanced stages of chronic kidney disease, preferably in collaboration with a multidisciplinary team, has been strongly recommended. Earlier referral provides the nephrologist time to identify and manage reversible conditions, ensure avoidance of nephrotoxic agents, administer specific therapies, recommend dietary and lifestyle changes to slow the progression of kidney decline, manage comorbidities and complications and institute regular follow-up, education and activation of social support. Even if progression to ESRD is inevitable, earlier nephrology care can optimally prepare the patient for renal replacement therapy, both physically and mentally. [12]

Researchers suggest that 12 months of pre-ESRD care by a specialist is optimal [12, 13].

As has been covered earlier, African American patient with ESRD and on dialysis have better outcomes than matched European American groups, but Kalbfleisch and colleagues looked at racial disparities in outcomes within almost 6000 dialysis facilities [14].

> Without race adjustment, facilities with higher proportions of black patients had better survival outcomes; facilities with the highest percentage of black patients (top 10%) had overall mortality rates approximately 7% lower than expected. After adjusting for within-facility racial differences, facilities with higher proportions of black patients had poorer survival outcomes among black and non-black patients; facilities with the highest percentage of black patients (top 10%) had mortality rates approximately 6% worse than expected. [14]

Essentially, the researchers contend that the better outcomes in African American predominant dialysis centers are misleading because they should actually be higher. It is only after adjusting for the better survival on dialysis by race, does these differences become evident.

Although poor access to healthcare, the APOL1 gene, and increased diabetes and hypertension greatly contribute to added renal disease in African Americans, well-designed studies have still failed to fully account for all of the excess kidney disease. Despite similar dietary sodium intake, renal handling, and plasma volume regulation, renal disease burden is substantially worse in African Americans compared to European Americans [15].

7.1   Hypertensive Nephrosclerosis

Persistent hypertension results in progressive kidney changes including arteriosclerosis, cortical fibrosis, tubular atrophy and loss, and glomerulosclerosis which is collectively referred to as hypertensive nephrosclerosis [16]. When compared to the majority population, African Americans have more severe nephrosclerosis, it begins at a younger age, and it results in renal failure more often [16]. The increased prevalence of hypertensive nephrosclerosis is principally attributed to the risk alleles associated with APOL1 and directly related to the increased burden of end-stage renal disease among African Americans [2, 3].

7.2   Obesity and Proteinuria

In addition to the genetic differences, researchers also suspect that obesity and its increased prevalence leading to diabetes in the African American community is driving up kidney disease [17]:

> We found that BMI was related independently to both urine total protein–creatinine and albumin-creatinine ratios, and that higher urine total protein–creatinine and urine albumin-creatinine ratios were observed in those with the highest BMI. This association was independent of traditional factors previously observed or hypothesized to be related to proteinuria, including BP, level of kidney function, glycemia, and hyperuricemia. In addition, we found that this association was particularly evident in individuals younger than 61 years. This finding raises the possibility that obesity is a risk factor for proteinuria and albuminuria in hypertensive nephrosclerosis and may have a role in the development and progression of kidney disease, particularly in younger patients. [17]

7.3   Kidney Disease Progression

In terms of tracking kidney disease progression, the African American Study of Kidney Disease and Hypertension (AASK) found that proteinuria (both baseline and follow-up) was a better predictor of subsequent kidney disease in African Americans than a baseline glomerular filtration rate (GFR) which is generally accepted as the best predictor [18]. In all, it is important to remember that measuring proteinuria is the most predictive in all racial and ethnic subgroups as a marker for renal disease.

Decreased education and low socioeconomic status have been shown to contribute to excess ESRD in African Americans [19, 20]. Other risk factors include:

- Male
- Diabetes history
- Smoking
- Hypertension

Despite the high prevalence and incidence of chronic and end-stage renal disease in African Americans, among those with kidney disease, African Americans have a better adjusted survival rate [19]. This paradox of improved survival in African Americans after initiation of dialysis has befuddled researchers given the disproportionate occurrence and increased comorbidities. Ma and colleagues at the Wake Forest School of Medicine suggest that the improved survival in nondiabetic-induced nephropathy may also be due to the very gene that causes the disparity, the APOL1 gene, but this time it conveys protection against further advancing atherosclerosis while on dialysis [21].

Time will sort out these genetic and phenotypic peculiarities, but the overall poor outcomes in renal disease persist, and their impact on the African American population remains clear and present.

7.4   Treatment and Counseling

As far as treatment, in contrast to the contraindications for the use of ACE inhibitors as a singular first line treatment of hypertension, the use of ACE inhibitors (and ARBs) is the mainstay of therapy for the reduction of adverse clinical outcomes for African American patients with kidney disease. Using an ACE or ARB in combination with a thiazide diuretic in African Americans with hypertensive nephrosclerosis has been shown to decrease the progression of disease [22]. Elevated blood pressure should be aggressively treated, and increased uric acid levels should be lowered.

Continued cigarette smoking also negatively impacts renal function, accelerates albuminuria, and decreases the glomerular filtration rate (GFR) in African Americans [23]. A large study of over 5000 participants found a dose-dependent (cigarette-per-day dependent) direct relationship with renal function decline and smoking: the more cigarettes per day, the faster the renal function decline. The study also found that smoking was also related to elevated CRP (C-reactive protein) levels suggesting that the smoking elevates inflammation in some way [23]. The more likely explanation links smoking and progressive vascular disease and worsened blood pressure control. Most patients with chronic kidney disease die of cardiovascular disease which speaks to the value of adequate hypertension control in patients with kidney disease, as well as persistent smoking cessation counseling [24, 25].

7.5   Kidney Transplantation

Finally, disparities also exist in kidney transplantation with fewer African American referrals for kidney transplantation [26]. Barriers to organ transplantation include African Americans' being less likely than European Americans to be supportive of organ donation [27], to be referred and evaluated for transplant [28], to be identified as a donor, and to consent to organ donation [28].

The issues related to African Americans consenting to organ donation have been the topic of much research, and the basis for skepticism in this sometimes life-saving process rests in cultural and experiential differences. Because African Americans have fewer transplants, the awareness in the community of successful and productive transplants remains low. It is important for many African American patients to understand that kidney donation does not require the sacrifice of life or that agreeing to other organ donations does not initiate a grand conspiracy to prematurely be declared dead for the benefit of others. The history of earned distrust of the medical community negatively impacts outcomes related to the donation and the receiving of life-saving organ transplantation. A study by Esther Brown at the School of Nursing at Widener University found five fundamental areas of "reluctance" to transplantation [27]:

1. A lack of awareness
2. Lack of trust of the medical profession
3. Fear of premature death
4. Racial discrimination
5. Religious beliefs and misconceptions

The overall decreased organ donation in the African American population decreases the options for closer genetic matches which can lead to better long-term graft survival. Another barrier is the increased comorbidities (diabetes and hypertension) in African Americans which may disqualify a potential African American donor. Families with members that have end-stage renal disease are frequently populated with others with the same problems, thus decreasing the pool of potential high-match living donors. Breakthroughs in genomic medicine have revealed that individuals with APOL1 genetic variants are associated with significantly decreased transplant graft survival [29]. Nephrologists have long known that kidneys from African American donors had significantly shorter allograft survival no matter the race of the recipient. In fact, African American recipients of non-African American kidneys have a higher likelihood of prolonged allograft survival [29].

Other African Americans simply disqualify themselves as potential donors due to a misperception of their own health and the thought that because of a history of poor dietary habits and lifestyle decisions, no one would want their organs [30].

Once kidney transplantation is indicated, several factors increase waiting time and negatively influence graft survival after transplantation. Outside of related donors, minimizing the genetic mismatches greatly improves transplant opportunity and ultimate success but naturally will negatively impact African American's waiting for the reasons discussed above. Having an African American donor or recipient negatively impacts graft survival for a number of factors that are poorly understood. Taber, Egede, and Baliga found a consistently higher rate of acute rejection and delayed graft function in African Americans with over 90% compromised after 5 years [31].

With a myriad of issues related to early diagnosis, occurrence, progression, preparation for dialysis, dialysis initiation, transplant planning, and post-transplant preservation, much work still needs to be done with African Americans and kidney disease.

7.6   Kidney Stones

Urinary tract calculi (kidney stones) are far more common in European Americans and Asians than in African Americans [32]. European American males are affected 3–4 times more often than African American males, though African Americans have a higher incidence of infected ureteral calculi than European Americans. The difference in the occurrence of stones between African American men and woman is small compared to the large difference based on sex in European Americans. African Americans tend to develop stones at an older age, and there is a curious but verified association with increased gall stones [33].

If an African American develops kidney stones, calcium oxalate and calcium phosphate stones are still the most common, but African Americans also have a higher propensity to form uric acid stones, have diabetes, and have a higher BMI and waist circumference. As part of the work-up for kidney stone, a 24-hour urine collection is a key aspect. Unfortunately, Eric Ghiraldi at the Einstein Healthcare Network found that "African American patients were half as likely to submit a 24-hour urine collection than (European American) patients" [34]. Spending more time describing the process, and purpose, of a 24-hour urine collection should improve your success with patient compliance.

Important Differences in Renal Disease

- There is at least a threefold increase in occurrence of renal disease among African Americans, but African Americans have a better adjusted survival rate.
- Diabetes and hypertension are generally the cause of ESRD in African Americans with nephropathy caused by renal-risk variants in the apolipoprotein L1 gene (*APOL1*).
- Vascular injury caused by smoking, obesity, diabetes, hyperlipidemia, and persistent hypertension accelerates kidney injury.
- Measuring proteinuria is the best way to tract kidney function in African Americans.
- African Americans should be advised of the one-to-one correlation between the amount of their cigarette smoking and their continued renal function decline.
- Kidney transplantation differences:
  - African Americans tend to be less open to donating organs for transplantation.
  - African Americans tend to be less aware of their options as related to kidney transplantation and also less aware of the specifics regarding the maintenance of a transplanted organ.
  - Kidney transplants in African Americans tend to have a shorter duration of viability.
  - Allograft survival is shorter in recipients of kidneys from African American donors relative to those donated by European Americans regardless of the race of the recipient.
- African Americans have a lower incidence of urinary tract calculi.
  - When they occur, African Americans have a *higher incidence* of infected ureteral calculi than European Americans.
  - When collecting a 24-hour urine sample, spend more time explaining the process and purpose for the collection.

References

1. Harding K, Mersha T, Webb F, Vassalotti J, Nicholas S. Current state and future trends to optimize the care of African Americans with end-stage renal disease. Am J Nephrol. 2017;46(2):156–64.
2. 2017 United States Renal Data System Annual Data Report: Executive Summary. https://www.usrds.org/2017/download/2017_Volume_1_CKD_in_the_US.pdf.

3. Sinha S, Shaheen M, Rajavashisth T, Pan D, Norris K, Nicholas S. Association of race/ethnicity, inflammation, and albuminuria in patients with diabetes and early chronic kidney disease. Diabetes Care. 2014;37(4):1060–8.

4. Parsa A, Kao W, Xie D, et al. APOL1 risk variants, race, and progression of chronic kidney disease. N Engl J Med. 2013;369(23):2183–96.

5. Freedman B, Limou S, Ma L, Kopp J. APOL1-associated nephropathy: a key contributor to racial disparities in CKD. Am J Kidney Dis. 72(5 Suppl 1):S8–S16.

6. Kruzel-Davila E, Wasser WG, Aviram S, Skorecki K. APOL1 nephropathy: from gene to mechanisms of kidney injury. Nephrol Dial Transplant. 2016;31(3):349–58.

7. Genovese G, Friedman DJ, Ross MD, Lecordier L, Uzureau P, Freedman BI, et al. Association of trypanolytic ApoL1 variants with kidney disease in African Americans. Science. 2010;329(5993):841–5.

8. Lertdumrongluk P, Streja E, Rhee CM, et al. Survival advantage of African American dialysis patients with end-stage renal disease causes related to APOL1. Cardiorenal Med. 2019;9(4):212–21.

9. African Americans and Kidney Disease. National Kidney Foundation. https://www.kidney.org/news/newsroom/factsheets/African-Americans-and-CKD. Accessed 10 May 2019.

10. Mehrotra R, Soohoo M, Rivara MB, Himmelfarb J, Cheung AK, Arah OA, et al. Racial and ethnic disparities in use of and outcomes with home dialysis in the United States. J Am Soc Nephrol: JASN. 2016;27(7):2123–34. Epub 2015/12/15. Eng.

11. Nee R, Moon DS, Jindal RM, et al. Impact of poverty and health care insurance on arteriovenous fistula use among incident hemodialysis patients. Am J Nephrol. 2015;42(4):328–36.

12. Gillespie BW, Morgenstern H, Hedgeman E, et al. Nephrology care prior to end-stage renal disease and outcomes among new ESRD patients in the USA. Clin Kidney J. 2015;8(6):772–80.

13. Norris KC, Williams SF, Rhee CM, et al. Hemodialysis disparities in African Americans: the deeply integrated concept of race in the social fabric of our society. Semin Dial. 2017;30(3):213–23.

14. Kalbfleisch J, Wolfe R, Bell S, et al. Risk adjustment and the assessment of disparities in dialysis mortality outcomes. J Am Soc Nephrol. 2015;26(11):2641–5.

15. Williams S, Ogedegbe G. Unraveling the mechanism of renin-angiotensin-aldosterone system activation and target organ damage in hypertensive blacks. Hypertension. 2011;59:10–1.

16. Hughson M, Puelles V, Hoy W, Douglas-Denton R, Mott S, Bertram J. Hypertension, glomerular hypertrophy and nephrosclerosis: the effect of race. Nephrol Dial Transplant. 2014;297(7):1399–409.

17. Lea J, Greene T, Hebert L, Lipkowitz M, Massry S, Middleton J, Rostand S, Miller E, Smith W, Bakris G. The relationship between magnitude of proteinuria reduction and risk of end-stage renal disease: results of the African American study of kidney disease and hypertension. Arch Intern Med. 2005;165(8):947–53.

18. Toto R. Lessons from the African American study of kidney disease and hypertension: an update. Curr Hypertens Rep. 2006;8(5):409–12.

19. Lipworth L, Mumma M, Cavanaugh K, Edwards T, Ikizler T, Tarone R, McLaughlin J, Blot W. Incidence and predictors of end stage renal disease among low-income blacks and whites. PLoS One. 2012;7(10):e48407.

20. Ward M. Socioeconomic status and the incidence of ESRD. Am J Kidney Dis. 2008;51(4):563–72.

21. Ma L, Langefeld C, Comeau M. APOL1 renal-risk genotypes associate with longer hemodialysis survival in prevalent nondiabetic African American patients with end-stage renal disease. Kidney Int. 2016;90(2):389–95.

22. Dirkx TC, Woodell T. Kidney disease. In: Papadakis MA, McPhee SJ, Rabow MW, editors. Current medical diagnosis & treatment; 2019. New York: McGraw-Hill. http://0-accessmedicine.mhmedical.com.crusher.neomed.edu/content.aspx?bookid=2449&sectionid=194574729. Accessed 11 May 2019.

23. Hall M, Wang W, Okhomina V, Agarwal M, Hall J, Dreisbach A, Juncos L, Winniford M, Payne T, Robertson R, Bhatnagar A, Young B. Cigarette smoking and chronic kidney disease in African Americans in the Jackson Heart Study. J Am Heart Assoc. 2016;5(6):e003280.

24. Rahman M, Pressel S, Davis B. Cardiovascular outcomes in high-risk hypertensive patients stratified by baseline glomerular filtration rate (GFR). Report from the Antihypertensive and Lipid-Lowering Treatment to Prevent Heart Trial (ALLHAT). Ann Intern Med. 2006;144(3):172–80.

25. Cheung A, Rahman M, Reboussin D, for the SPRINT Research Group. Effects of intensive blood-pressure control in CKD. J Am Soc Nephrol. 2017;28:2812–23. ISSN: 1046-6673/2809.

26. Kumar K, Holscher C, Luo X, Wang J, Anjum S, King E, Massie A, Tonascia J, Purnell T, Segev D. Persistent regional and racial disparities in nondirected living kidney donation. Clin Transpl. 2017;31(12):e13135.

27. Brown E. African American present perceptions of organ donation: a pilot study. ABNF J. 2012;23(2):29–33.

28. Sieverdes J, Nemeth L, Magwood G, Baliga P, Chavin K, Ruggiero K, Treiber F. African American kidney transplant patients' perspective on challenges in the living donation process. Prog Transplant. 2015;25(2):164–75.

29. Freedman B, Julian B. Should kidney donors be genotyped for APOL1 risk alleles? Kidney Int. 2015;87(4):671–3.

30. DuBay D, Ivankova N, Herby I, Wynn T, Kohler C, Berry B, Foushee H, Carson A, Redden D, Holt C, Siminoff L, Fouad M, Martin M. African American organ donor registration: a mixed methods design using the theory of planned behavior. Prog Transplant. 2014;24(3):273–83.

31. Taber D, Egede L, Baliga P. Outcome disparities between African Americans and Caucasians in contemporary kidney transplant recipients. Am J Surg. 2017;213(4):666–72.

32. Akoudad S, Szklo M, McAdams M, Fulop T, Anderson C, Coresh J, Kottgen A. Correlates of kidney stone disease differ by race in a multi-ethnic middle aged population: the ARIC study. Prev Med. 2010;51(5):416–20.

33. Ahmed M, Barakat S, Almobarak A. The association between renal stone disease and cholesterol gallstones: the easy to believe and not hard to retrieve theory of the metabolic syndrome. Ren Fail. 2014;36(6):957–62.

34. Ghiraldi E, Reddy M, Li T, Lawler A, Friedlander J. Factors associated with compliance in submitting 24-hour urine collections in an underserved community. J Endourol. 2017;31(S1):S64–8.

Important Differences in Rheumatic Diseases

8

Mobility disability as manifested as arthritis and other rheumatic disorders are the leading causes of physical disability in the United States. The proportion impacted increases as poverty increases with African Americans disproportionately comprising this group. There are important considerations when treating African Americans patients with rheumatic diseases in particular, and some can make a significant impact in terms of early diagnosis and morbidity aversion [1].

In contrast to osteoarthritis which is conventionally viewed as a result of "wear and tear," rheumatic disorders comprise an array of autoimmune-mediated diseases including:

- Rheumatoid arthritis
- Systemic lupus erythematosus
- Ankylosing spondylitis and psoriatic arthritis
- Sjögren syndrome
- Scleroderma
- Polymyalgia rheumatica and giant cell arteritis

There has been a significant debate regarding whether African Americans express autoimmune diseases differently than other racial/ethnic groups and whether these differences are genetically mediated or related to the social determinants of health. Does the disproportionate occurrence of systemic lupus erythematosus in African American women, in particularly a greater risk of progression to end-stage renal disease and dialysis, relate somehow to their innate immune function? Or is the immune response related to the stresses of living a life of poverty, social pressure, and racism? The outcomes are clear: African Americans have more severe cases of

© Springer Nature Switzerland AG 2020
G. L. Hall, *Patient-Centered Clinical Care for African Americans*,
https://doi.org/10.1007/978-3-030-26418-5_8

immune-mediated diseases overall. The exact causes for these adverse outcomes are still being investigated.

Early-life socioeconomic disadvantage has become increasingly targeted as a lasting social determinant of health [2]. Data in rheumatologic studies across the spectrum of diseases suggest that childhood low socioeconomic status increases the risk of later disease [3–6].

While the mystery of increased autoimmune disorders in African Americans will remain essentially a modern day "nature versus nurture" debate, clinicians have to treat the patients in front of them including their social determinants, and African Americans with immune-mediated diseases will require specialized attention.

8.1   Osteoarthritis

Osteoarthritis (OA) is a multifactorial joint disease characterized by cartilage degradation and structural changes in the subchondral bone, which often leads to joint pain, activity limitations, and physical disability. Middle-aged and older African Americans experience disproportionate rates of functional limitations and disabilities from osteoarthritis when compared to other racial/ethnic groups [7–9]. Specifically, African Americans report greater pain and activity limitation than European Americans. Although researchers have suggested that these disproportionate rates of functional limitations in African Americans may be due to increased obesity rates, poor physical activity, and decreased tolerance of pain in general, it remains unclear what other factors may be related to this disparity [10].

Jordan and colleagues at the Thurston Arthritis Research Center at the University of North Carolina found that "African Americans had a slightly higher prevalence of knee symptoms, radiographic knee OA, and symptomatic knee OA, but a significantly higher prevalence of severe radiographic knee OA compared to (European Americans)" [11].

The Johnston County Osteoarthritis Project in Durham, North Carolina, looked at knee, hip, and multiple joint outcomes and found that "African Americans and (European Americans) with only hip OA or both hip and knee OA did not differ in self-reported pain or function." But the study did find differences in patients with only knee OA and attributed the difference to increased BMI (obesity) and the presence of depression. The authors suggested improving the management of obesity and depressive symptoms as key avenues to successful management of osteoarthritis pain [12]. This Project also found distinct differences in common foot disorders with flat feet (pes planus) being three times more common in African Americans and high arches (pes cavus) being five times less common [13]. African Americans were also more likely to have bunions (hallux valgus), hammer toes, and overlapping toes [13].

Vaughn et al. did a meta-analysis comparing pain from osteoarthritis in European Americans and African Americans, and their review confirmed differences in clinical pain severity, functional limitations, and poor performance between African Americans and European Americans with osteoarthritis [14, 15].

Burns et al. added another confounding layer to the OA debate by reporting that frequently African American and European Americans "with radiographically documented knee OA reported equivalent functional ability and pain severity. However, both (African Americans)'s OA severity rating and tested performance were significantly worse than those of (European Americans)" [16].

Despite some suggestion of a genetic variant that makes OA of the knee different in African Americans, the consensus seems to be that overall osteoarthritis is fairly similar across races/ethnicities but the perceptions of pain, mobility, and impact on activities of daily living are different [14].

8.2 Rheumatoid Arthritis

Rheumatoid arthritis (RA) is a chronic systemic disease associated with progressive joint damage and inflammation, diminished quality of life, significant disability, and premature mortality. In contrast to a number of chronic diseases where there is no doubt in the worse outcomes in African Americans, there is more controversy regarding the existence of disparities in RA. When objective clinical signs like rheumatoid nodules, joint deformities on radiographs, and tender joints are considered, there seems to be fewer differences between racial and ethnic groups [17]. In contrast, functional status in African Americans with RA generally shows decreased abilities and lower ranking of self-reported health when compared to majority populations [18].

In a review of laboratory trends, African American RA patients tended to have rheumatoid factor positive results in slightly more cases (80% of patients) compared to European Americans (74% of patients) [18].

In all patients with RA, early joint damage (within the first few years) is highly predictive of more damaging disease later and a clear indicator of the need for more aggressive treatment in all patients [19]. Advancing these patients to "disease-modifying antirheumatic drugs" (DMARDs) including hydroxychloroquine, sulfasalazine, methotrexate, and other newer options can slow progression and prevent deformities. Unfortunately, remission rates on DMARDs were comparatively lower in African Americans but still significantly beneficial [18].

8.3   Systemic Lupus Erythematosus

Systemic lupus erythematosus (SLE) is a chronic autoimmune disease which effects an array of organ systems including diffuse joint involvement, dermatitis, pleuritis, myocarditis, hepatitis, blood dyscrasias, and nephritis. African American woman have a three- to fourfold increased presentation of SLE when compared to European American woman, and like other chronic diseases have increased morbidity and mortality related to the disease [20]. SLE can present in a number of unusual fashions. So unusual that experts suggest that if you have an African American woman with a number of seemingly unrelated symptoms that wax and wane, a screen for SLE is a very reasonable diagnostic approach.

SLE Presentation
- Low-grade fever
- Malaise and fatigue
- Weight changes
- Sun-sensitive rash (malar rash)
- Arthritis effecting two or more joints
- Oral ulcers (painless)
- Pleuritis
- Proteinuria
- Seizures or psychosis
- Headaches
- Premature atherosclerosis
- Anemia
- Low WBC
- Low platelet count

Gender disparities also exist with SLE occurring far more often in women (8–10 times more prevalent than in men) [20, 21].

A number of studies have confirmed a much more severe disease course in African Americans with an earlier onset, higher incidence of kidney failure, progression to dialysis, and kidney transplant complications. Lymphadenopathy is also a common feature with an increased risk of progression to lymphoma. Arthritis is seen in 95% of SLE patients and frequently involves the wrists and hands [20, 22, 23]. Kidney involvement in the form of nephritis is the most common manifestation in SLE and is seen microscopically in over 90% of patients but results in significant disease in 50% of patients [24, 25]. The APOL1 gene that results in increased kidney disease in African Americans (see Chap. 7) makes SLE-related kidney disease much more severe. This gene is so intertwined with renal decline that receiving a transplanted kidney from a donor with the APOL1 gene makes recurrent kidney failure more common [26, 27].

A study by Franco and colleagues looked at predictors of kidney failure in African Americans and found that hypertension, elevated creatinine, proliferative nephritis, and decreased GFR were all associated with an increased risk [27]. Another investigator found that hypertension and proteinuria significantly impacted the SLE disease course in African Americans [28].

There have also been significant investigations into environmental influences on SLE. Carroll et al. did an extensive evaluation of environmental exposures including water analysis, diet, lifestyle factors (smoking and pesticide use), industry proximity, soil chemical data, and more and statistically matched the presence, or development, of antinuclear antibodies (ANA) [29]. Increased exposure to pollutants positively correlated with increased occurrences of ANA status and SLE development. Unfortunately, African Americans are disproportionately exposed and impacted.

As far as treatment differences between races with SLE, none existed. There were indications that vitamin D supplementation may be useful in African American patients with SLE when decreased vitamin D levels were found when compared to controls [30–32].

In terms of behaviors contributing to increased SLE risk, the Black Women's Health Study and others found that smoking increases the risk of developing the disease, whereas moderate alcohol consumption was associated with decreased risk [33–36].

Patients with systemic lupus erythematosus have a high prevalence of hypertension, accelerated atherosclerosis, and arterial stiffness that substantially increases their risk for a cardiovascular-related death [37, 38]. SLE itself carries an independent risk for coronary artery disease even after adjustment for traditional Framingham risk factors [39]. Risk analyses for perioperative medical management of SLE patients show an increased risk for cardiac and venous thromboembolism in patient with total knee or hip replacement. These patients also had higher perioperative infections suggesting the need for withdrawing immunosuppressive medications earlier [40].

SLE-associated chronic immune-mediated inflammation and damage to the arterial walls causes aortic stiffness, which then leads to hypertension, which then promotes atherosclerosis. Studies have confirmed higher aortic stiffness in younger SLE patients that seem to be independent of age, blood pressure, renal function, and risk factors. In fact, SLE patients with normal blood pressure had consistently higher aortic stiffness [41].

As reviewed earlier, SLE can be tricky to diagnose as it can affect any organ including musculoskeletal, skin, hematologic, renal, neuropsychiatric, cardiovascular, and respiratory system. There is no typical order of presentation aside from fatigue and arthritis pain being pervasive complaints. Another clue is increased healthcare utilization in the form of higher than expected emergency department or urgent care visits. SLE should also be suspected in any patient who presents with unexplained manifestations involving two or more organ systems [42].

Glucocorticoids and antimalarial drugs form the foundation of SLE management along with immunosuppressive medications and newer biologic therapies. As the pathogenesis of SLE becomes clearer, more targeted, and better tolerated, treatments will become available [43].

8.4   Ankylosing Spondylitis

Ankylosing spondylitis (AS) is a debilitating spinal arthritic condition usually presenting before age 40, with male predominance, and a very low presentation in African Americans when compared to other racial groups. AS can present with acute uveitis, peripheral arthritis, enthesitis, psoriasis, aortic root inflammation, and gut irritation. Ankylosing spondylitis involves both inflammatory erosive osteopenia and unusual bony overgrowth [44]. The major histocompatibility complex (MHC) class I allele human leukocyte antigen B27 (HLA-B27) accounts for the majority of the genetic risk for ankylosing spondylitis. The prevalence of HLA-B27 varies widely between ethnic populations, with an approximate 8–10% prevalence in European Americans and much lower 2–4% in African Americans [45].

8.5   Primary Sjögren's Syndrome

Sjögren's syndrome is a chronic, slowly progressing autoimmune disease characterized by lymphocytic infiltration of the exocrine glands resulting in xerostomia and dry eyes. The majority of patients with Sjögren's syndrome have symptoms related to impaired tear formation and salivary gland function. The disease progression is slow and a majority of patients manage well. Like ankylosing spondylitis and polymyalgia rheumatica, this has a rare presentation in African Americans [46, 47].

8.6   Scleroderma (Systemic Sclerosis)

Scleroderma, also known as systemic sclerosis (SSc), is a chronic disorder characterized by diffuse fibrosis of the skin and internal organs. Women are affected four times more frequently than men [48]. Scleroderma had a modestly higher prevalence among African Americans than European Americans. In most patients the impact is limited to the face, neck, and extremities; however some patients have more severe and wide-ranging involvement. Raynaud's phenomenon is frequently present, but GERD, pulmonary fibrosis, pulmonary hypertension, and renal problems occur as well. Raynaud's phenomenon generally precedes other disease manifestations and may be the presenting complaint. CREST syndrome is an acronym for scleroderma's common associated problems including calcinosis cutis, Raynaud's phenomenon, esophageal dysmotility, sclerodactyly, and telangiectasia.

African Americans generally have more severe manifestations of scleroderma, and the aggressiveness of the disease seems to be linked to socioeconomic status. Higher SES African Americans have a milder disease, whereas poorer patients tend to have a more complicated course [49].

Duncan Moore, Virginia Steen and colleagues at Georgetown University Hospital looked at scleroderma in a large retrospective evaluation of clinical outcomes by race. They found that African Americans with scleroderma tend to have worse disease outcomes with more severe pulmonary disease with increased fibrosis noted on imaging as well as decreased overall lung function [48]. Worse cardiac disease with increased pulmonary hypertension on right heart catheterization was also noted in African Americans [50]. African American patients are more likely to have the confirmatory markers, anti-Scl70 (anti-topoisomerase) and anti-U1RNP antibodies, than European American patients. They were less likely to have anti-centromere antibodies than majority populations. Overall, African Americans tended to be younger at disease onset and were hospitalized more frequently. Interestingly, their study found that after controlling for socioeconomic status, "African American race was not a statistically significant independent mortality risk factor and that a lower household income increased the risk of death during follow-up" [48].

The differences seen in Scleroderma are not based on race but instead based on a social determinant of health. The opportunity to completely erase the significant disparities seen in scleroderma is completely within our reach [51].

8.7   Polymyalgia Rheumatica and Giant Cell Arteritis

Polymyalgia rheumatica (PMR) is an inflammatory condition that generally affects people over the age of 50 and can cause profound pain and stiffness in the proximal muscles of the shoulders, neck, and hip. Giant cell arteritis (GCA), or temporal arteritis, is an inflammatory disease affecting the large blood vessels of the scalp, neck, and arms which causes a narrowing of the blood vessels. Polymyalgia rheumatica and giant cell arteritis probably represent a spectrum of one disease: one localized and the other more systemic [52]. The vasculitic involvement of these arteries leads to the typical symptoms of GCA such as temporal headache, jaw pain, scalp tenderness, or abnormal temporal arteries on biopsy. Both affect the same older population, and the incidence increases with advancing age. Women are effected two to three times more often than men. PMR and giant cell arteritis is distinctly less common in Asian, African American, and Latino/Hispanic populations, though all racial and ethnic groups can be affected [53]. Both PMR and GCA respond well to steroid administration.

8.8   Gout

Gout is the most common inflammatory arthritis in the United States and is more common in African Americans principally due to a higher prevalence of risk factors [54]. The increased incidence of diabetes, obesity, hypertension, and chronic kidney disease in African Americans contributes to higher uric acid levels which directly increase the risk for gout attacks. African American diet trends that increase the risk for hyperuricemia include:

- Increased meat consumption which leads to excess purine that is degraded to uric acid
- Increased sugary-sweetened beverages, whereby fructose metabolism leads to increased uric acid levels
- Decreased vitamin C-containing fruits and vegetables lead to decreased uric acid clearing
- Less overall alcohol consumed but when used, leads to increased uric acid production [54]

The disorders usually associated with gouty attacks are clinically time-consuming chronic diseases including coronary artery disease, diabetes, kidney disease, and hypertension. In comparison, these more life-threatening diseases supplant gout complaints and any discussion of strategies for improvement in the uric acid. Studies have shown that reducing uric acid levels has been associated with better overall outcomes including lower cardiovascular mortality and slowed kidney failure [55].

A number of studies have documented lower uric acid levels in younger African Americans (average age 24 in one case) when compared to European Americans, but after maturity their low risk disappears [56]. Aside from diet, the environmental, genetic, and physiologic factors explaining the uric acid differences between African Americans and European Americans remain obscure. Uric acid excretion abnormalities are the most common causes of hyperuricemia and make sense considering comorbidities seem to drive some of the increased risk [57].

Given the increased comorbidities, choosing the right medications can be a challenge. Hydrochlorothiazide is suggested as first line for the treatment of hypertensive African Americans yet also well-known to increase uric acid levels [58, 59]. Furthermore, a study at Johns Hopkins found that metoprolol increased the serum uric acid in African Americans with kidney disease that were treated for hypertension [60]. The researchers found no increase with ACE inhibitors or amlodipine [60]. This basically leaves amlodipine as the lone best choice for treating African Americans with hypertension, renal insufficiency, and a risk for gout. It is well accepted that hyperuricemia is a risk factor for kidney disease progression, given its increased occurrence in African Americans; the uric acid level should be used as a risk screen even in the absence of gout attacks [61]. In addition, the use of allopurinol has been suggested to slow the progression of renal disease.

Lifestyle Modifications for African Americans with High Uric Acid and/or Gout
- Lose weight
- Avoid fructose-containing sugary-sweetened beverages
- Limit red meat (beef, pork, and lamb) and seafood
- Limit certain vegetables including potatoes, spinach, asparagus, peas, cauliflower, and mushrooms
- Avoid alcohol (particularly beer and liquor)
- Increase dairy intake (eggs, low fat milk, yogurt cheese) if not lactose intolerant
- Get regular exercise

Overall the treatment of gout in African Americans is no different than any other racial group or ethnicity. Patients should be counseled regarding dietary and behavioral modifications first. Suggestions should be specific. African Americans should avoid fructose-containing sugary-sweetened beverages ("high fructose corn syrup") [54]. Red meat (beef, pork, and lamb) and seafood should be significantly limited. Certain vegetables also lead to higher uric acid levels including potatoes, mushrooms, spinach, asparagus, cauliflower, and peas [54, 62]. Remember to assess the patient's alcohol intake, recommend a decrease, and particularly discourage beer [62]. Daily intake of coffee has been shown to be protective of gout [63], as has vitamin C and cherry juice [64]. Although there is increased lactose intolerance in African Americans, those not intolerant should increase their dairy intake in the form of skim milk, cheese, and eggs [62, 66]. A study by Dalbeth and colleagues found a decrease in uric acid levels of 10% in those that consumed milk [65]. Like in many disorders related to lifestyle habits, exercise and weight loss are always beneficial [66].

Important Differences in Rheumatological Disease
- Racial differences exist in clinical pain severity, functional limitations, and poor performance between African Americans and European Americans with osteoarthritis, but the differences are small.
- Data in rheumatologic studies across the spectrum of diseases suggest that childhood low socioeconomic status increases the risk of later life disease.
- Flat feet (pes planus) is three times more common in African Americans, while high arches (pes cavus) is five times less common. African Americans were also more likely to have bunions (hallux valgus), hammer toes, and overlapping toes.
- African American RA patients tended to have rheumatoid factor positive results in slightly more cases (80% of patients) compared to European Americans (74% of patients).
- The APOL1 gene that results in increased kidney disease in African Americans makes SLE-related kidney disease much more severe.
- In all patients with RA, early joint damage (within the first few years) is very predictive of more damaging disease later and a clear indicator of the need for more aggressive treatment.
- Patients with SLE and hypertension, higher creatinine, and decreased GFR are at higher risk for dialysis.
- There is an environmental exposure and SLE outcome relationship such that the occurrence and severity of SLE are more prominent in urban industrial regions.
- The APOL1 gene results in increased and earlier kidney disease progression in African Americans with SLE.
- Patients with SLE and hypertension, higher creatinine, proliferative nephritis, and decreased GFR as well as genetic, environmental, and socioeconomic factors were associated with increased ESRD requiring dialysis.
- Ankylosing spondylitis (AS) is a debilitating spinal arthritic condition related to HLA-B27 which is found in 2–4% of African Americans.
- Sjögren's syndrome is a chronic, slowly progressing autoimmune disease that rarely occurs in African Americans.

- Scleroderma had a modestly higher prevalence among African Americans than European Americans.
- African Americans generally have more severe manifestations of scleroderma, and the aggressiveness of the disease seems to be linked to socioeconomic status. Higher SES African Americans have a milder disease, whereas poorer patients tend to have a more complicated course.
- Both PMR and GCA rarely occur in African Americans.
- African Americans start with a lower risk for gout but, as they age, develop a higher risk due to dietary, environmental, genetic, and physiologic factors.
- Hydrochlorothiazide increases the risk for hyperuricemia.
- Metoprolol increases the risk for hyperuricemia in African Americans with chronic kidney disease.

References

1. Okoro CA, Hollis ND, Cyrus AC, Griffin-Blake S. Prevalence of disabilities and health care access by disability status and type among adults — United States, 2016. MMWR Morb Mortal Wkly Rep. 2018;67:882–7. https://doi.org/10.15585/mmwr.mm6732a3External.
2. Kamp Dush CM, Schmeer KK, Taylor M. Chaos as a social determinant of child health: reciprocal associations? Soc Sci Med. 2013;95:69–76.
3. Brennan SL, Turrell G. Neighborhood disadvantage, individual-level socioeconomic position, and self-reported chronic arthritis: a cross-sectional multilevel study. Arthritis Care Res (Hoboken). 2012;14(5):721–8.
4. Cleveland RJ, Schwartz TA, Prizer LP, Randolph R, Schoster B, Renner JB, Jordan JM, Callahan LF. Associations of educational attainment, occupation, and community poverty with hip osteoarthritis. Arthritis Care Res (Hoboken). 2013;14(6):954–61.
5. Bengtsson C, Nordmark B, Klareskog L, Lundberg I, Alfredsson L. Socioeconomic status and the risk of developing rheumatoid arthritis: results from the Swedish EIRA study. Ann Rheum Dis. 2005;14(11):1588–94.
6. Morgan Banks L, Kuper H, Polack S. Poverty and disability in low- and middle-income countries: a systematic review. PLoS One. 2017;12(12):e0189996.
7. Allen KD, Helmick CG, Schwartz TA, DeVellis RF, Renner JB, Jordan JM. Racial differences in self-reported pain and function among individuals with radiographic hip and knee osteoarthritis: the Johnston County osteoarthritis project. Osteoarthr Cartil. 2009;17(9):1132–6.
8. Burns R, Graney MJ, Lummus AC, Nichols LO, Martindale-Adams J. Differences of self-reported osteoarthritis disability and race. JAMA. 2007;99(9):1046–51.
9. Andresen EM, Brownson RC. Disability and health status: ethnic differences among women in the United States. J Epidemiol Community Health. 2000;54(3):200–6.
10. Colbert CJ, Almagor O, Chmiel JS, Song J, Dunlop D, Hayes KW, Sharma L. Excess body weight and four-year function outcomes: comparison of African Americans and whites in a

prospective study of osteoarthritis. Arthritis Care Res (Hoboken). 2013;65(1):5–14. https://doi.org/10.1002/acr.21811.

11. Jordan JM, Helmick CG, Renner JB, et al. Prevalence of knee symptoms and radiographic and symptomatic knee osteoarthritis in African Americans and Caucasians: the Johnston County Osteoarthritis Project. J Rheumatol. 2007;34(1):172–80.

12. Allen KD, Helmick CG, Schwartz TA, et al. Racial differences in self-reported pain and function among individuals with radiographic hip and knee osteoarthritis: the Johnston County Osteoarthritis Project. Osteoarthr Cartil. 2009;17(9):1132–6.

13. Golightly Y, Hannan MT, Dufour AB, Jordan JM. Racial differences in foot disorders and foot type. Arthritis Care Res (Hoboken). 2012 Nov;64(11):1756–9.

14. Vaughn IA, Terry EL, Bartley EJ, et al. Racial-ethnic differences in osteoarthritis pain and disability: a meta-analysis. J Pain. 2019;20:629–44. Pii: S1526-5900(18)30964-7.

15. Cruz-Almeida Y, Sibille KT, Goodin BR, et al. Racial and ethnic differences in older adults with knee osteoarthritis. Arthritis Rheumatol. 2014;66(7):1800–10.

16. Burns R, Graney M, Lummus AC, et al. Differences of self-reported osteoarthritis disability and race. J Natl Med Assoc. 2007;99(9):1046–51.

17. Mikuls TR, Kazi S, Cipher D, et al. The association of race and ethnicity with disease expression in male US veterans with rheumatoid arthritis. J Rheumatol. 2007;34(7):1480–4.

18. Greenberg JD, Spruill T, Shan Y, et al. Racial and ethnic disparities in disease activity in rheumatoid arthritis patients. Am J Med. 2013;126(12):1089–98.

19. Bridges SL, Causey ZL, Burgos PI, et al. Radiographic severity of rheumatoid arthritis in African Americans: results from the CLEAR Registry. Arthritis Care Res (Hoboken). 2010;62(5):624–31.

20. Williams EM, Bruner L, Adkins A, et al. I too, am America: a review of research on systemic lupus erythematosus in African Americans. Lupus Sci Med. 2016;3(1):e000144.

21. Harley JB, Kelly JA. Genetic basis of systemic lupus erythematosus: a review of the unique genetic contributions in African Americans. J Natl Med Assoc. 2002;94(8):670–7.

22. Barbhaiya M, Feldman CH, Guan H, et al. Race/ethnicity and cardiovascular events among patients with systemic lupus erythematosus. Arthritis Rheumatol. 2017;69(9):1823–31.

23. Burgos PI, McGwin G Jr, Pons-Estel GJ, et al. US patients of Hispanic and African ancestry develop lupus nephritis early in the disease course: data from LUMINA, a multiethnic US cohort (LUMINA LXXIV). Ann Rheum Dis. 2011;70:393–4.

24. Alarcón GS, Bastian HM, Beasley TM, et al. Systemic lupus erythematosus in a multi-ethnic cohort (LUMINA) XXXII: [corrected] contributions of admixture and socioeconomic status to renal involvement. Lupus. 2006;15:26–31.

25. Contreras G, Lenz O, Pardo V, et al. Outcomes in African Americans and Hispanics with lupus nephritis. Kidney Int. 2006;69:1846–51.

26. Freedman BI, Limou S, Ma L, Kopp JB. APOL1-associated nephropathy: a key contributor to racial disparities in CKD. Am J Kidney Dis. 2018 Nov;72(5S1):S8–S16.

27. Franco C, Yoo W, Franco D, et al. Predictors of end stage renal disease in African Americans with lupus nephritis. Bull Hosp Jt Dis. 2010;68:251–6.

28. Lea JP. Lupus nephritis in African Americans. Am J Med Sci. 2002;323:85–9.

29. Carroll R, Lawson AB, Voronca D, et al. Spatial environmental modeling of autoantibody outcomes among an African American population. Int J Environ Res Public Health. 2014;11:2764–79.

30. Ravenell R, Kamen D, Spence J, et al. Premature atherosclerosis is associated with hypovitaminosis D and angiotensin-converting enzyme inhibitor non-use in lupus patients. Am J Med Sci. 2012;344:268–73.

31. Hoffecker BM, Raffield LM, Kamen DL, Nowling TK. Systemic lupus erythematosus and vitamin D deficiency are associated with shorter telomere length among African Americans: a case-control study. PLoS One. 2013;8(5):e63725.

32. Word AP, Perese F, Tseng LC, et al. 25-Hydroxyvitamin D levels in African-American and Caucasian/Hispanic subjects with cutaneous lupus erythematosus. Br J Dermatol. 2012;166:372–9.

33. Formica MK, Palmer JR, Rosenberg L, et al. Smoking, alcohol consumption, and risk of systemic lupus erythematosus in the Black Women's Health Study. J Rheumatol. 2003;30:1222–6.

34. Cozier YC, Barbhaiya M, Castro-Webb N, et al. Relationship of cigarette smoking and alcohol consumption to incidence of systemic lupus erythematosus in the Black Women's Health Study. Arthritis Care Res (Hoboken). 2018;71:671. https://doi.org/10.1002/acr.23703.

35. Kiyohara C, Wasakazu M, Horiuchi T, et al. Cigarette smoking, alcohol consumption, and risk of systemic lupus erythematosus: a case-control study in a Japanese population. J Rheumatol. 2012;39(7):1363–70.

36. Takvorian SU, Merola JF, Costenbader KH. Cigarette smoking, alcohol consumption and risk of systemic lupus erythematosus. Lupus. 2014;23(6):537–44.

37. Becker-Merok A, Nossent J. Prevalence, predictors and outcome of vascular damage in systemic lupus erythematosus. Lupus. 2009;18:508–15.

38. Liang MH, Mandl LA, Costenbader K, et al. Atherosclerotic vascular disease in systemic lupus erythematosus. J Natl Med Assoc. 2002;94:813–9.

39. Esdaile JM, Abrahamowicz M, Grodzicky T, et al. Traditional Framingham risk factors fail to fully account for accelerated atherosclerosis in systemic lupus erythematosus. Arthritis Rheum. 2001;44(10):2331–7.

40. Goodman SM, Bass AR. Perioperative medical management for patients with RA, SPA, and SLE undergoing total hip and total knee replacement: a narrative review. BMC Rheumatol. 2018. https://doi.org/10.1186/s41927-018-0008-9.

41. Roldan CA, Joson J, Qualls CR, et al. Premature aortic stiffness in systemic lupus erythematosus by transesophageal echocardiography. Lupus. 2010;19(14):1599–605.

42. Pramanik B. Diagnosis of systemic lupus erythematosus in an unusal presentation: what a primary care physician should know. Curr Rheumatol Rev. 2014;10(2):81–6.

43. Sciascia S, Rdin M, Roccatello D, et al. Recent advances in the management of systemic lupus erythematosus. F1000Res. 2018;7.

44. Smith JA. Update on ankylosing spondylitis: current concepts in pathogenesis. Current concepts in pathogenesis. Curr Allergy Asthma Rep. 2015;15:489.

45. Kopplin LJ, Mount G, Suhler EB. Review for disease of the year: epidemiology of HLA-B27 associated ocular disorders. Ocul Immunol Inflamm. 2016;24(4):470–5.

46. Helmick CG, Felson DT, Lawrence RC, et al. Estimates of the prevalence of arthritis and other rheumatic conditions in the United States: part 1. Arthritis Rheum. 2008;58(1):15–25.

47. Brito-Zerón P, Acar-Denizli N, Zeher M, on behalf of the EULAR-SS Task Force Big Data Consortium, et al. Influence of geolocation and ethnicity on the phenotypic expression of primary Sjögren's syndrome at diagnosis in 8310 patients: a cross-sectional study from the Big Data Sjögren Project Consortium. Ann Rheum Dis. 2017;76:1042–50.

48. Moore DF, Kramer E, Eltaraboulsi R, Steen VD. Increased morbidity and mortality of scleroderma in African Americans compared to non-African Americans. Arthritis Care Res. 2019;71(9):1154–63.

49. Gelber AC, Manno RL, Shah AA, et al. Race and association with disease manifestations and mortality in scleroderma: a 20-year experience at the Johns Hopkins Scleroderma Center and review of the literature. Medicine (Baltimore). 2013;92(4):191–205.

50. McNearney TA, Reveille JD, Fischbach M, Friedman AW, Lisse JR, Goel N, et al. Pulmonary involvement in systemic sclerosis: associations with genetic, serologic, sociodemo-graphic, and behavioral factors. Arthritis Rheum. 2007;57:318–26.

51. Morgan ND, Gelber AC. African Americans and scleroderma: examining the root cause of the association. Arthritis Care Res (Hoboken). 2019;71:1151. https://doi.org/10.1002/acr.23860.

52. Gonzalez-Gay MA, Matteson EL, Castaneda S. Polymyalgia rheumatica. Lancet. 2017;390(10103):1700–12.

53. Smith CA, Fidler WJ, Pinals RS. The epidemiology of giant cell arteritis. Report of a ten-year study in Shelby County, Tennessee. Arthritis Rheum. 1983;26(10):1214–9.

54. Kumar B, Lenert P. Gout and African Americans: reducing disparities. Cleve Clin J Med. 2016;83(9):665–74.

55. Karis E, Crittenden DB, Pillinger MH. Hyperuricemia, gout, and related comorbities: cause and effect on a two-way street. South Med J. 2014;107:235–41.

56. Gaffo AL, Jacobs DR Jr, Lewis CE, Mikuls TR, Saag KG. Association between being African-American, serum urate levels and the risk of developing hyperuricemia: findings from the coronary artery risk development in young adults cohort. Arthritis Res Ther. 2012;14:R4.

57. Juraschek SP, Kovell LC, Miller ER, Gelber AC. Gout, urate-lowering therapy, and uric acid levels among adults in the United States. Arthritis Care Res. 2015;67(4):588–92.

58. Wright J, Probstfield JL, Cushman W, et al. ALLHAT findings revisited in the context of subsequent analyses, other trials, and meta-analyses. Arch Intern Med. 2009;169(9):832–42.

59. Musini VM, Nazer M, Bassett K, Wright JM. Blood pressure-lowering efficacy of monotherapy with thiazide for primary hypertension. Cochrane Database Syst Rev. 2014;(5):CD003824.

60. Juraschek SP, Appel LJ, Miller ER. Metoprolol increases uric acid and risk of gout in African Americans with chronic kidney disease attributed to hypertension. Am J Hypertens. 2017;30(9):871–5.

61. Kumagai T, Ota T, Tamura Y, et al. Time to target uric acid to retard CKD progression. Clin Exp Nephrol. 2017;21(2):182–92.

62. Major TJ, Topless RK, Albeth N, Merriman TR. Evaluation of the diet wide contribution to serum urate levels: meta-analysis of population based cohorts. BMJ. 2018;363:k3951.

63. Park KY, Kim HJ, Ahn HS, et al. Effects of coffee consumption on serum uric acid: systematic review and meta-analysis. Semin Arthritis Rheum. 2016;45(5):580–6.

64. Martin KR, Coles KM. Consumption of 100% tart cherry juice reduces serum urate in overweight and obese adults. Curr Dev Nutr. 2019;3(5):nzz011.

65. Dalbeth N, Wong S, Gamble GD, et al. Acute effect of milk on serum urate concentrations: a randomized controlled crossover trial. Ann Rheum Dis. 2010 Sep;69(9):1677–82.

66. Richette P, Doherty M, Pascual E, et al. 2016 updated EULAR evidence-based recommendations for the management of gout. Ann Rheum Dis. 2017;76(1):29–42.

Important Differences in Pulmonary Diseases

Disparities in outcomes for pulmonary diseases are the most evident of all chronic diseases. A "Disparities in Respiratory Health" report put out jointly by the American Thoracic Society, and the European Respiratory Society indicates that "the lowest social groups are up to 14 times more likely to have respiratory diseases than the highest" [1]. Some data also suggests that African Americans may be more susceptible to chronic lung disease due to a smaller trunk/leg ratio compared to European Americans [2, 3]. The relatively smaller thorax in African Americans (and woman) may make exposure to toxins, like cigarette smoke, more damaging with less exposure. Other possible explanations include genetic/epigenetic differences, proteases, and/or cytokines that may influences how the lung reacts to exposures [2].

9.1   COPD (Emphysema and Chronic Bronchitis)

While COPD has historically been considered a "white male smoker's disease," newer data and migrating smoking demographics have shown an increased prevalence in woman and a rapidly growing incidence in African Americans. Chronic obstructive pulmonary disease (COPD) disproportionately affects ethnic minorities and low socioeconomic groups not just in the United States but across the world. Because of disproportional poverty and urban living, African Americans have an increased exposure to indoor and outdoor pollution, occupational and environmental hazards, and tobacco smoke, which contribute to disparities in prevalence and outcomes of COPD. In short, the social determinants of health (healthcare access, educational opportunities, economic stability, and social and community environment) complicate the course of COPD for too many African Americans [3].

© Springer Nature Switzerland AG 2020   109
G. L. Hall, *Patient-Centered Clinical Care for African Americans*,
https://doi.org/10.1007/978-3-030-26418-5_9

Although African Americans are thought to have an overall lower prevalence of COPD in the United States, several reports have demonstrated that African Americans develop COPD with less cumulative smoking and at younger ages [4, 5]. These worse outcomes are more pronounced in the presence of current smoking, asthma, maternal smoking, and maternal COPD. Data suggests that the prevalence of emphysema is lower in African Americans while chronic bronchitis is higher when compared by race (Fig. 9.1).

Chronic Bronchitis – Prevalence Rates per 1,000, 2011

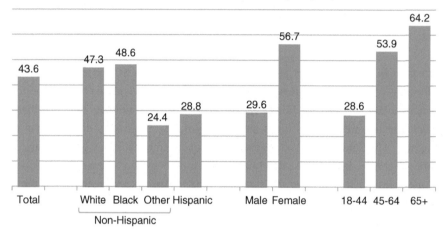

Source: CDC. NHIS 2011.

Emphysema – Prevalence Rates per 1,000, 2011

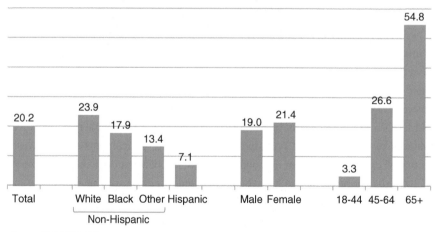

Source: CDC. NHIS 2011.

Fig. 9.1 Prevalence of chronic bronchitis and emphysema by race, sex, and age. https://www. lung.org/assets/documents/research/copd-trend-report.pdf

A study by Hardin et al. at Harvard Medical School showed that African Americans had a significantly higher history of asthma and therefore were more likely to have more frequent COPD exacerbations [6].

COPD is an independent risk factor for lung cancer, with chronic bronchitis and/ or emphysema increasing lung cancer risk by two- to fivefold as compared to smokers with normal spirometry. African Americans are at higher risk for developing COPD and lung cancer [7]. Research done by Mark Dransfield showed that African Americans (women in particular) are more susceptible to the damaging effects of tobacco smoke when compared to European American men [8]. Therefore, while all tobacco smokers may be at comparable risk for the development of COPD, African Americans and women who develop COPD may be particularly susceptible to progressive disease [9, 10]. These added adverse events make smoking cessation counseling critical.

Another study by Han et al. looked at quality of life and related it to COPD exacerbations and found that African Americans had more frequent hospitalizations despite similar quality of life indexes [11]. The same study noted disparities in home oxygen prescriptions, influenza vaccination administrations, and referral for smoking cessation counseling which were surmised to be contributing to the increased hospitalizations [11].

Hyun Lee and colleagues looked at NHANES data for COPD-related comorbidities to see if racial differences existed and found some interesting trends [12]. African Americans had a number of comorbidities including a high prevalence of current smokers, a history of asthma, hypertension, stroke, diabetes, anemia, and rheumatoid arthritis [12].

Finally, Tadahiro Goto at Massachusetts General looked at the readmission rates for patients with COPD. Overall there was a 20% 30-day readmission rate for patients with COPD. When examined by race, he found that African American patients had a higher rate of asthma-COPD overlap with asthma as a predominant cause for readmission. COPD patients with asthma had significantly more exacerbations and readmissions. Because of the asthma component, the authors presumed that long-acting beta2-agonist and inhaled corticosteroid use would benefit these patients more [13]. When African American patients present with COPD, it is critical to determine if they have a history of asthma.

9.2 Asthma

Asthma occurs in almost 14% of African American children with a higher prevalence in girls (15.7% compared to 11.4%) [14]. African American adults are three times more likely to die from asthma. In fact, mortality rates are highest in African

American women, whose rate is more than two times higher than that of European American women. African American children have a death rate ten times that of European American children [14]. Overall, the African American mortality rate, emergency department visit rate, and hospital admission rate for asthma are all multiple times higher than European Americans [15]. Despite the high mortality, increased ED visits and hospitalizations, and poor outcomes, African Americans have lower physician office visits, lower specialty office visits, and lower levels of asthma care as recommended by guidelines [16]. Because of the fewer referrals to pulmonologists, there is less pulmonary function testing and diagnosis confirmation. Given the worse outcomes yet less intensive interventions, front-line providers have a unique opportunity to make a big difference in the quality of care of asthma in this population.

Risk factors for increased mortality in patients with asthma include multiple emergency department visits or hospitalizations, history of intubation or ICU admission in the past 5 years, non-use of inhaled corticosteroids, current smoking, psychosocial stress and depression, socioeconomic factors, and negative attitudes and beliefs regarding the benefit of medications [15]. Unfortunately, African Americans disproportionately have these comorbidities, factors, and beliefs.

As in COPD, environmental factors also play a prominent role in the frequency and severity of asthma. Because African Americans live disproportionately in urban areas where industrial pollutants and occupational exposures occur, asthma occurrence and severity are worse. Differences in housing, with a higher rate of living in poverty, also increase the exposure to asthma-inducing antigens (dust, dust mites, mold, cockroaches, mice, rats, and more). Rates of asthma were also significantly higher among children whose home exteriors and interiors were described as being in "poor condition" [17]. Essentially, social and economic variables working at the individual, household, and neighborhood level can greatly impact the occurrence and severity of asthma [18].

Obesity is another important modifiable risk factor. Higher BMI is associated with more uncontrolled asthma, increased severity of asthma, and increased number of medications. Weight loss is associated with improved outcomes [19]. Addressing obesity and its impact on asthma with our patients is important.

A study by Brehm et al. at Brigham and Woman's Hospital found that vitamin D deficiency was associated with increased asthma severity [20]. The vitamin D insufficiency occurred more often with older age, higher BMI, and African American race. When the vitamin D level exceeded 30 ng/ml, the likelihood of an asthma exacerbation decreased. The odds of any hospitalization or emergency department visit was higher in patients with low vitamin D even after adjusting for age, sex, BMI, and baseline asthma severity [20]. A majority of African Americans have low vitamin D levels [21]. Note that a number of other researchers have also looked at the connection between vitamin D and asthma and not found either a true connection, or benefit from vitamin D supplementation [22].

Another curious finding was the positive association with breast feeding and a lower prevalence of asthma exacerbations, even after controlling for socioeconomic status, maternal smoking, BMI, and a number of other factors [23]. One third of African American children are never breast fed and are also at increased risk for worse asthma outcomes [23].

The treatment of asthma is essentially the same across racial groups with a long-acting beta2-agonist and inhaled corticosteroid combination resulting in greater improvements in pulmonary function and asthma control [14].

9.3 Sarcoidosis

Sarcoidosis is a multisystem disease of unknown origin characterized by non-caseating granulomatous inflammation at the affected site. Although any organ can be involved, the disease most commonly (>90%) affects the lungs and intrathoracic lymph nodes. Disparities in outcomes exist by race, ethnicity, sex, and socioeconomic groups, with African Americans having disproportionately more severe disease. Mortality rates are highest in African Americans, and they tend to have more severe lung involvement [24–26]. Environmental exposures are also linked to sarcoidosis due to a clustering of outbreaks during flu seasons. Geographic variations with increased occurrences in the southeast and coastal areas also support a role for environmental factors in sarcoidosis. Some scientists suggest that exposure to molds, mildews, and musty odors at home or work conveys a small increased risk [27].

It remains unclear how much racial differences are due to genetics, socioeconomic factors, or a combination of the two. Researchers have found specific genes in African Americans that are associated with more severe disease and worse outcomes and another set of genes in European Americans that are associated with milder disease [28]. Data show that lower socioeconomic status patients have more advanced and persisting disease with African Americans comprising a greater proportion of these patients [29].

Sarcoidosis is more often symptomatic in African Americans and has more extrapulmonary presentations including more skin, bone marrow, and eye involvement when compared to majority populations. Even the lung involvement is more obvious with African American patients having decreased forced vital capacity and increased shortness of breath. African Americans have higher granuloma density compared with other races despite similar stages of disease and are diagnosed approximately 10 years earlier than European American patients, due to earlier onset of symptoms [29].

A study by Mirsaeidi and colleagues of mortality in patients with sarcoidosis found dramatically more deaths due to respiratory failure, cardiac arrest, pulmonary hypertension, heart failure, pulmonary fibrosis, hypertension, diabetes, and renal failure [29]. Overall African Americans had an eightfold higher mortality rate compared to European Americans. This study also found a different geographical distribution for African Americans with increased cases in the District of Columbia, North and South Carolina, Pennsylvania, and New Jersey [29].

There are also differences in outcomes based on ethnicity and gender among families with sarcoidosis with African American women dying at a higher rate and younger age than European Americans. Yvette Cozier and colleagues at the Slone Epidemiology Center at Boston University looked closely at sarcoidosis in African American women as part of the Black Women's Health Study [25]:

> the lung was the organ most commonly involved in the disease process, with 61% of women having lung involvement, followed by intrathoracic lymph nodes (35%); 96% had intrathoracic involvement. There was also substantial extrapulmonary disease; sites affected most often were the skin (including erythema nodosum) (20%), and eyes (16%). Cardiac sarcoidosis was reported for only one woman. Chest radiograph was reported as the method of diagnosis for 73% of women, followed by biopsy (54%), and chest CT scan (31%). Sixty percent of women with a diagnostic chest radiograph were classified by their physicians as stage II or higher. Comorbid illness was noted for 56% of cases: conditions reported by physicians included asthma, hypertension, type 2 diabetes, cancer, scleroderma, lupus, obesity, hypercholesterolemia, and depression. [25]

In terms of clinical presentation, patients in this study presented with shortness of breath (45%), fatigue (41%), and cough (40%) most frequently [25]. Twenty-five percent presented with sinus congestion and 20% had chest pain. Palpitations as a presenting complaint are highly suggestive of sarcoid cardiac involvement [30]. Pulmonary hypertension, which occurs more often in African Americans, heralds a poor prognosis when developed [31, 32].

There is general consensus that patients with sarcoidosis and no evidence of end-organ impairment and minimal respiratory symptoms should not be treated [33]. Because African Americans tend to have more severe disease with more varied organ involvement, it is going to be critical that these patients be followed closely. If more advanced disease is determined, the treatment generally involves steroids for an extended period of time. Steroid-sparing medications (hydroxychloroquine, methotrexate, azathioprine, tumor necrosis factor, etc.) are also gaining popularity, but no studies related to response differences based on race have indicated any advantages [33].

9.4   Obstructive Sleep Apnea (OSA)

A study by Chen et al. at the Harvard School of Public Health confirmed there are more sleep apnea, interrupted sleep, and daytime sleepiness in African Americans than in European Americans [33]. The lost sleep leads to daytime sleepiness, fatigue, poor concentration, poor energy, increased hypertension, heart disease, poor digestion and metabolism, and more [34].

A number of studies have found increased sleep-disordered breathing in African Americans, and these disparities persist even after controlling for BMI [35–37]. While increased obesity does directly increase the occurrence of OSA in African Americans, it is likely not the entire cause. In terms of risk factors, African Americans tend to have craniofacial soft tissue features that contribute to obstructive sleep apnea including a larger tongue area. For those significantly obese patients, weight loss can reverse obstructive sleep apnea in some [38].

There is also a significant disparity with African American children having 20% more sleep apnea severity and oxygen desaturation [35].

African American children are 4-6 times more likely to have OSA compared to white children. Even among young adults less than 26 years of age, African Americans are 88% more likely to have OSA as compared to whites. Among middle-aged populations, the evidence for a disparity in OSA prevalence is weaker as differences in OSA prevalence from community based studies are evident in some but not all studies. In contrast, data from older populations suggests a disparity may re-emerge in this age group. While African Americans had similar prevalence of OSA as whites (32% and 30% respectively) in a community-based survey of individuals 65 years of age and older, this group was 2.1 times more likely to have severe OSA. [35]

Chen also found significantly increased sleep apnea patterns with more snoring, more obesity, and worse global functioning in African Americans. They also showed decreased formally diagnosed sleep apnea in African Americans despite the disproportional increased occurrence [34].

African Americans have a poorer sleep quality overall associated with shortest sleep duration and the highest levels for excessive daytime sleepiness [39]. With prolonged loss of sleep, the risk for hypertension and resultant strokes, heart disease, and kidney failure ensues [40].

Continuous positive airway pressure (CPAP) therapy is the treatment of choice for mild, moderate, and severe obstructive sleep apnea. CPAP reduces daytime sleepiness, depression, and hypertension and improves alertness and global quality of life [41].

Schwartz and colleagues at the University of South Florida looked at veteran data and found that only a fraction of patients with sleep apnea and a CPAP machine use it. In African Americans, the use of this technology is even worse. African Americans were over five times more likely to not use their CPAP machine than European Americans [42]. They also found that when African Americans had severe OSA, they were three times more likely to use CPAP than African Americans with mild or moderate symptoms [42].

Addressing poor compliance with CPAP usage has been a growing medical concern. Jessie Bakker and colleagues at Harvard Medical School looked at an array of published approaches to improved compliance with CPAP and concluded that remote monitoring associated with a personalized behavioral modification plan would likely be part of the solution to this difficult and pervasive problem [43].

> To be implemented clinically, it is critical that an adjunct therapy to promote CPAP adherence be cost-effective, feasible in a wide range of settings, and scalable to large and diverse patient populations. The most efficacious interventions tested to date have been behavioral in nature; when combined with the remote-monitoring capabilities available in modern CPAP machines, these theory-driven methods could hold the answer to increasing real-world CPAP adherence rates. [43]

Patients with sleep apnea will need a compliance discussion on follow-up visits that includes an assessment of their CPAP comfort including mask style, sleeping position, and what approaches they have used to improve compliance. It is also worth reviewing the significant improvement in sleep apnea comorbidities (hypertension, cardiovascular, daytime alertness, etc.) when emphasizing CPAP use.

Important Differences in Pulmonary Diseases
- Because of disproportional poverty and urban living, African Americans have an increased exposure to indoor and outdoor pollution, occupational and environmental hazards, and tobacco smoke, which contribute to disparities in prevalence and outcomes of COPD.
- African American patients had a higher rate of asthma-COPD overlap with asthma as a predominant cause for resistant treatment and hospital readmission.
- African Americans have a higher rate of chronic bronchitis and a lower rate of emphysema when compared to European Americans.
- Vitamin D insufficiency is associated with higher odds of severe asthma exacerbation, and having a vitamin D level greater than 30 ng/ml is protective against severe asthma exacerbations.

- African Americans with COPD are significantly younger, smoke less, report concurrent asthma more frequently, and have less radiographic emphysema on volumetric computed tomography.
- There is more sleep apnea, interrupted sleep, and daytime sleepiness in African Americans than in European Americans.
- African Americans had a significantly higher history of asthma and were more likely to have more frequent COPD exacerbations.
- African Americans (women in particular) are more susceptible to the damaging effects of tobacco smoking when compared to European American men.
- Asthma occurs in almost 14% of African American children with a higher prevalence in girls.
- African American mortality rate, emergency department visit rate, and hospital admission rate for asthma are all multiple times higher than European Americans.
- Obesity is associated with more uncontrolled asthma, increased severity of asthma, and increased number of medications.
- Breast feeding is associated with a lower prevalence and severity of asthma.
- Sarcoidosis is more severe (eight times higher mortality) with more end-organ damage in African Americans with an increased occurrence in woman.
- African Americans have a poorer sleep quality overall associated with worse insomnia levels and the highest levels for excessive daytime sleepiness.
- African Americans were over five times more likely to not use their CPAP machine than European Americans.

References

1. Schraufnagel DE, Blasi F, Kraft M, et al. An official American Thoracic Society/European Respiratory Society policy statement: disparities in respiratory health. Am J Respir Crit Care Med. 2013;188(7):865–71.
2. Staton GW, Ochoa CD. Chronic obstructive pulmonary disease. In: McKean SC, Ross JJ, Dressler DD, Scheurer DB, editors. Principles and practice of hospital medicine. 2nd ed. New York: McGraw-Hill. http://0-accessmedicine.mhmedical.com.crusher.neomed.edu/content.aspx?bookid=1872&sectionid=146988856. Accessed 12 June 2019.
3. Pleasants RA, Riley IL, Mannino DM. Defining and targeting health disparities in chronic obstructive pulmonary disease. Int J Chron Obstruct Pulmon Dis. 2016;11:2475–96.

4. Chatila WM, Wynkoop WA, Vance G, Criner GJ. Smoking patterns in African Americans and whites with advanced COPD. Chest. 2004;125(1):15–21.
5. Foreman MG, Zhang L, Murphy J, et al. Early-onset chronic obstructive pulmonary disease is associated with female sex, maternal factors, and African American race in the COPD Gene Study. Am J Respir Crit Care Med. 2011;184:414–20.
6. Hardin M, Silverman EK, Barr RG, et al. The clinical features of the overlap between COPD and asthma. Respir Res. 2011;12:127. https://doi.org/10.1186/1465-9921-12-127.
7. Mina N, Soubani AO, Cote ML, et al. The relationship between COPD and lung cancer in African American patients. Clin Lung Cancer. 2012;13(2):149–56.
8. Dransfield MT, Davis JJ, Gerald LB, Bailey WC. Racial and gender differences in susceptibility to tobacco smoke among patients with chronic obstructive pulmonary disease. Respir Med. 2006;100(6):1110–6.
9. Kirkpatrick dP, Dransfield MT. Racial and sex differences in chronic obstructive pulmonary disease susceptibility, diagnosis, and treatment. Curr Opin Pulm Med. 2009;15(2):100–4.
10. Kamil F, Pinzon I, Foreman MG. Sex and race factors in early-onset COPD. Curr Opin Pulm Med. 2013;19(2):140–4.
11. Han MK, Curran-Everett D, Dransfield MT, et al. Racial differences in quality of life in patients with COPD. Chest. 2011;140(5):1169–76.
12. Lee H, Shin SH, Gu S, et al. Racial differences in comorbidity profile among patients with chronic obstructive pulmonary disease. BMC Med. 2018;16:178.
13. Goto T, Faridi MK, Gibo K, et al. Sex and racial/ethnic differences in the reason for 30-day readmission after COPD hospitalization. Respir Med. 2017;131:6–10.
14. Asthma and African Americans. U.S. Department of Health and Human Services Office of Minority Health. 2018. https://minorityhealth.hhs.gov/omh/browse.aspx?lvl=4&lvlid=15. Accessed 12 June 2019.
15. Brown RW, Cappelletti CS. Reaching beyond disparity: safely improving asthma control in the at-risk African American population. J Natl Med Assoc. 2013;105(2):138–49.
16. Krishnan JA, Diette GB, Skinner EA, et al. Race and sex differences in consistency of care with national asthma guidelines in managed care organizations. Arch Intern Med. 2001;161(13):1660–8.
17. Holt EW, Theall KP, Rabito FA. Individual, housing, and neighborhood correlates of asthma among young urban children. J Urban Health. 2013;90(1):116–29.
18. Bruzzese JM, Kingston S, Falletta KA, et al. Individual and neighborhood factors associated with undiagnosed asthma in a large cohort of urban adolescents. J Urban Health. 2019;96(2):252–61.
19. Loman DG, Kwong CG, Henry LD, et al. Asthma control and obesity in urban African American children. J Asthma. 2017;54(6):578–83.
20. Brehm JM, Schuemann B, Fuhlbrigge AL, et al. Serum vitamin D and severe asthma exacerbations in the childhood asthma management program study. J Allergy Clin Immunol. 2010;126(1):52–56.e5.
21. Harris SS. Vitamin D and African Americans. J Nutr. 2006;136(4):1126–9.

22. Hall SC, Agrawal DK. Vitamin D and bronchial asthma: an overview of the last five years. Clin Ther. 2017;39(5):917–29.

23. Oh S, Du R, Zeiger AM, et al. Breastfeeding associated with higher lung function in African American youths with asthma. J Asthma. 2017;54(8):856–65.

24. Gerke AK, Judson MA, Cozier YC, et al. Disease burden and variability in sarcoidosis. Ann Am Thorac Soc. 2017;14(Suppl 6):S421–8.

25. Cozier YC, Berman JS, Palmer JR, Boggs DA, Serlin DM, Rosenberg L. Sarcoidosis in black women in the United States: data from the Black Women's Health Study. Chest. 2011;139:144–50.

26. Gideon NM, Mannino DM. Sarcoidosis mortality in the United States 1979–1991: an analysis of multiple-cause mortality data. Am J Med. 1996;100:423–7.

27. Newman LS, Rose CS, Bresnitz EA, ACCESS Research Group, et al. A case control etiologic study of sarcoidosis: environmental and occupational risk factors. Am J Respir Crit Care Med. 2004;170:1324–30.

28. Levin AM, Adrianto I, Datta I, et al. Association of HLA-DRB1 with sarcoidosis susceptibility and progression in African Americans. Am J Respir Cell Biol. 2015;53(2):206–16.

29. Mirsaeidi M, Machado RF, Schraufnagel D, et al. Racial difference in sarcoidosis mortality in the United States. Chest. 2015;147(2):438–49.

30. Mehta D, Lubitz SA, Frankel Z, et al. Cardiac involvement in patients with sarcoidosis: diagnostic and prognostic value of outpatient testing. Chest. 2008;133(6):1426–35.

31. Judson MA, Boan AD, Lackland DT. The clinical course of sarcoidosis: presentation, diagnosis, and treatment in a large white and black cohort in the United States. Sarcoidosis Vasc Diffuse Lung Dis. 2012;29:119–27.

32. Rabin DL, Richardson MS, Stein SR, Yeager H. Sarcoidosis severity and socioeconomic status. Eur Respir J. 2001;18:499–506.

33. Beegle SH, Barba K, Gobunsuy R, Judson MA. Current and emerging pharmacological treatments for sarcoidosis: a review. Drug Des Devel Ther. 2013;7:325–38.

34. Chen X, Wang R, Zee P, et al. Racial/ethnic differences in sleep disturbances: the Multi-Ethnic Study of Atherosclerosis (MESA). Sleep. 2015;38(6):877–88.

35. Dudley KA, Patel SR. Disparities and genetic risk factors in obstructive sleep apnea. Sleep Med. 2016;18:96–102.

36. Ruiter ME, DeCoster J, Jacobs L, Lichstein KL. Sleep disorders in African Americans and Caucasian Americans: a meta-analysis. Behav Sleep Med. 2010;8(4):246–59.

37. Scharf SM, Seiden L, DeMore J, Carter-Pokras O. Racial differences in clinical presentation of patients with sleep-disordered breathing. Sleep Breath. 2004;8:173–83.

38. Joosten SA, Khoo JK, Edwareds BA, et al. Improvement in obstructive sleep apnea with weight loss in dependent on body position during sleep. Sleep. 2017;40(5):zsx047. https://doi.org/10.1093/sleep/zsx047.

39. Hayes AL, Spilsbury JC, Patel SR. The Epworth score in African American populations. J Clin Sleep Med. 2009;5:344–8.

40. Jhamb M, Unruh M. Bidirectional relationship of hypertension with obstructive sleep apnea. Curr Opin Pulm Med. 2014;20(6):558–64.

41. Epstein LJ, Kristo D, Strollo PJ Jr, et al. Clinical guideline for the evaluation, management and long-term care of obstructive sleep apnea in adults. J Clin Sleep Med. 2009;5(3):263–76.
42. Schwartz SW, Sebastiao Y, Rosas J, et al. Racial disparity in adherence to positive airway pressure among US veterans. Sleep Breath. 2016;20(3):947–55.
43. Bakker JP, Weaver TE, Parthasarathy S, Aloia MS. Adherence to CPAP: what should we be aiming for, and how can we get there? Chest. 2019;155(6):1272–87.

Important Differences in Hematology Results and Hematological Diseases

Before dealing with the few hematological diseases that are different in African Americans, it makes sense to review the hematology laboratory differences that exist between African American patients and majority patients. Many providers struggle with the decisions that need to be made when laboratory test results are outside of the normal range. Slightly lower or higher than reference range results can sometimes lead to follow-up laboratory tests, unnecessary referrals, and unwarranted investigations. Laboratory reference interval differences by race (and gender) have been recognized for many years, but clinical laboratories have been slow to adopt either race- or gender-linked reference ranges [1].

10.1 Laboratory Results

In a report by the Mayo Clinic, 60–70% of clinical decisions regarding a patient's diagnosis, treatment, hospital admission, and discharge were based on laboratory results [2]. Clinicians also "routinely experience uncertainty and challenges in ordering and interpreting diagnostic laboratory tests" [3]. Traditionally, reference intervals used in clinical laboratories have been determined using predominantly European American reference individuals. However, variances in reference range values have routinely been noted between racial/ethnic groups. Despite many calls for reference ranges tailored for racial specification, aside from "GFR African American and GFR Non-African American," laboratories continue to report a single "majority" reference range. Below is a consolidation of the adjustments and trends that should be considered when interpreting an African American patient's laboratory report.

© Springer Nature Switzerland AG 2020   121
G. L. Hall, *Patient-Centered Clinical Care for African Americans*,
https://doi.org/10.1007/978-3-030-26418-5_10

10.2 CBC

Eunjung Lim and colleagues at the Office of Biostatistics and Quantitative Health Sciences at the University of Hawaii looked at the reference intervals for common clinical laboratory results and found significant differences in gender and racial/ethnic subpopulations that could impact decision-making. Compared to European Americans, the normal range for African Americans significantly shifted to lower values in hemoglobin (HGB), hematocrit (HCT), mean corpuscular hemoglobin (MCH), and mean corpuscular hemoglobin concentration (MCHC) [4]. A number of studies have also shown lower total white blood cell (CBC) counts, neutrophil count, monocyte count, and platelet counts in African Americans when compared to European Americans [5–9].

CBC Trends in African Americans

WBC	*Lower*
HGB	*Lower*
HCT	*Lower*
MCH	*Lower*
MCHC	*Lower*
Neutrophils	*Lower*
Monocytes	*Lower*
Lymphocytes	*Higher*
Eosinophils	*Same*
Platelet count	*Lower*

10.3 Benign Ethnic Neutropenia

The asymptomatic reduction in white blood cell counts is principally driven by decreased neutrophil counts and has been seen in a number of racial groups but occurs most frequently in African Americans. Benign ethnic neutropenia (defined as between 1.0×10^9 cell/Liter and 1.5×10^9 cell/Liter) has increased prevalence in patients with genetic roots in North Africa, the Middle East, and South Asia [10]. Many healthy African Americans with low neutrophil counts undergo costly investigations, as well as delayed treatment, for a condition that has been demonstrated to be completely benign. Matthew Hsieh and colleagues looked at NHANES data and noted statistically significant differences in neutropenia by race. One in 22 African American men and 1 in 40 African American women have benign ethnic neutropenia [6]. In sharp contrast, European Americans have a neutropenia prevalence of 1 in 126.

The low neutrophil counts were tracked to a specific chromosome containing a receptor that influenced white blood cell production, and particularly neutrophils, in African Americans [11]. Rahul Lakhotia from the National Institute of Health looked at this phenomenon and "confirmed that the clinical nature for this condition was benign" [11]. The patients in his review with low neutrophil counts actually had low rates of infections as well as lower chronic disorders including hypertension and diabetes [11].

Benign ethnic neutropenia usually follows a hereditary pattern, and so a more detailed family history in neutropenic patients may reveal this cause [12, 13].

Patients with benign ethnic neutropenia do not require extensive monitoring or evaluation once this is discovered and incorporated into their past medical history. Otherwise if incidentally discovered, repeat the absolute neutrophil count three times within an interval of 2 weeks looking for count variations or signs/symptoms of infection. When determining the need for a diagnostic evaluation for neutropenia, clinicians should consider the patient's age, sex, and ethnicity [13, 14].

10.4   Metabolic Panel

Houman Tahmasebi and Khosrow Adeli of the CALIPER Program in Toronto, Canada, looked at the influence of ethnicity on population laboratory reference values and its impact on care [15]:

> Using RIs (reference intervals) established from a predominantly Caucasian population to interpret laboratory test results from a non-Caucasian or multi-ethnic patient population may lead to inaccurate interpretation of test results and, ultimately, missed diagnosis. For example, creatine kinase (CK) is commonly used as a biomarker for monitoring statin-induced myopathy to determine whether an individual can safely undergo or continue statin therapy. The median CK activity for healthy Black adult males and females is approximately double that of Caucasian adult males and females, respectively. The lack of an appropriate ethnic-specific RI for Black patients could result in termination of statin treatment in the absence of muscle toxicity, simply because their CK levels are above a RI established using a predominantly Caucasian reference population. In the absence of robust RIs that are ethnic-specific, clinicians are not able to provide the best possible healthcare for all patients. [15]

Laboratory Trends in African Americans

TSH	*Lower*
CRP	*Higher*
Creatine kinase (CK)	*Higher*
Creatinine	*Higher*
GGT	*Higher*
Total protein	*Higher*
Transferrin	*Lower*
PTH	*Higher*

When considering the general electrolytes, a number of studies have shown no significant difference in sodium, potassium, chloride, calcium, phosphorus, or magnesium between African Americans and European Americans [16].

10.5   Thyroid-Stimulating Hormone (TSH)

Laura Boucai at Albert Einstein College of Medicine looked at thyroid-stimulating hormone (TSH) in European Americans, African Americans, and Mexican Americans from NHANES data and found statistically significant differences in "normal" reference ranges for these racial/ethnic groups [17]. In general, African Americans have lower TSH levels with a range of 0.37–3.46 mIU/L (compared to "overall" reference interval 0.512–5.22 mIU/L) [17]. When a lower TSH level is found, this may prompt follow-up laboratory investigations (e.g., T3 and T4) and the additional costs involved. A simple understanding that African Americans have a lower reference interval for TSH can be reassuring and save time and money.

10.6   Lipid Profile

As is mentioned in the cardiovascular section, the lipid profile in African Americans is generally more favorable with a higher HDL and lower total cholesterol, LDL, and triglycerides [18]. This seemingly better profile is in stark contrast to worse cardiovascular outcomes for African Americans and should be considered when deciding who needs cholesterol-lowering medications and what criteria is used.

Lipid Profile Trends in African Americans	
Total cholesterol	*Lower*
HDL	*Higher*
LDL	*Lower*
Triglyceride	*Lower*

10.7   Cancer Markers

As reviewed in the cancer chapter, the prostate-specific antigen (PSA) is a better and more sensitive detector of prostate cancer in African Americans [19]. PSA also tends to range higher in cancer-free African Americans [20]. Veda Giri at Fox Chase

Cancer Center in Philadelphia PA found that at any given PSA, African Americans are at a higher risk for prostate cancer than European Americans. For example, a PSA of 3 gives a higher risk for prostate cancer to an African American than a matched European American with the same PSA [21]. The increased prostate cancer risk supports the need to follow "accelerating" PSAs, one that is rising over time yet still within normal limits, more closely in African Americans as this pattern is more associated with prostate cancer diagnosis [22]. PSA velocity, as it is also called, predicted more aggressive prostate cancer and a higher risk for death in African Americans [22]. In contrast, the study also found that PSA velocity did not add any significant utility over static PSA testing in European Americans or Asian Americans [22, 23].

Cancer Markers in African Americans	
PSA	*Higher*

10.8 Vitamins

The vitamin level differences in African Americans, with the exception of vitamin D, which is related to sun exposure and skin pigmentation, have largely been attributed to dietary differences [24–27]. Clinicians have correctly chosen to supplant these deficiencies with vitamin replacement. Multiple investigations have tracked low vitamin levels from childhood in African Americans, and while some believe this is linked to a lower socioeconomic status, larger studies have verified race/ethnicity as the strongest independent predictor [28]. It has been suggested that racial/ethnic differences in serum vitamin B-12 and folate concentrations may reflect race differences in bioavailability and metabolism of these nutrients, but replacement is still indicated [28].

Vitamin Level Trends in African Americans	
Vitamin B6	*Lower*
Vitamin B12	*Higher*
Vitamin C	*Higher*
Vitamin D	*Lower*
Vitamin E	*Lower*
Folate	*Lower*

10.9   Sickle Cell Disease

Sickle cell disease (SCD) is an inherited hemoglobinopathy and is the most common genetic blood disorder in the world. Sickled erythrocytes cause blood flow obstruction, hemolysis, and several hemostatic changes that promote coagulation. These events, in turn, induce chronic inflammation, which promote a hypercoagulable state which can cause the downstream complications including end-organ compromise [29].

Like the protection afforded by apolipoprotein L1 gene (APOL1) to African sleeping sickness while conferring an increased risk for kidney failure, sickle cell anemia offered a survival advantage in African regions where malaria was prevalent. The exact process for how a sickle-shaped cell results in less malarial disease burden is still the topic of much debate, but there is no question that prior to the development of antimalarial medications, having sickle cell anemia afforded a competitive advantage to those individuals. After migration to the Americas, the selective advantage of sickle cell anemia was lost as the exposure to malaria was erased.

The Centers for Disease Control and Prevention (CDC) now estimates that sickle cell anemia occurs in 1 in 365 African American births. Sickle cell trait, the heterozygous presentation, affects 1 in 13 African Americans who usually have symptom-free lives. Emerging evidence, however, is pointing to an increased risk for kidney disease and a reduction in GFR in patients with sickle cell trait [30].

More than two million Americans are estimated to be either heterozygous or homozygous for sickle cell. Most of those affected are of African ancestry, but a minority are of Hispanic or Southern European, Middle Eastern, or Asian Indian descent.

Complications are common among those with sickle cell disease and occur throughout the lifespan. The sickle cell inflammatory response can cause occlusion of arterial vessels which result in ischemia of the organs' supplied. The ischemia leads to severe pain. These recurrent acute vaso-occlusive crises are the most common manifestation of sickle cell disease and the most common reason for hospital admission.

Chronic complications of sickle cell disease may occur as a result of repeated acute episodes. Several of the most common of the chronic complications like chronic pain, cognitive loss due to stroke, renal dysfunction, splenic infarction, pulmonary hypertension, and retinal problems cause a significant degree of suffering.

The hallmark of the successful management of any disease is the prevention of complications. In sickle cell disease, preventing infections is critical. All patients should be vaccinated against *Streptococcus pneumoniae* and should be instructed to seek immediate attention whenever an infection is likely (fever >101 F) [31].

10.9.1 Renal Complications

Renal abnormalities manifested as sickle cell nephropathy can start with defects in urine concentration and acidification beginning in early childhood and progress with age to microalbuminuria, overt proteinuria, glomerulosclerosis, and, in some people, renal failure. Screening for albumin and protein in the urine to detect early decline in function is critical [32]. When albumin and protein suggest kidney function compromise in patients with sickle cell disease, angiotensin-converting enzyme (ACE) inhibitors have shown great value [32].

10.9.2 Pulmonary Hypertension

Pulmonary hypertension, which is an elevation of the pulmonary arterial pressure, occurs frequently in patients with sickle cell disease. When sickle cell disease patients present with shortness of breath, dyspnea on exertion, fatigue, palpitations, chest pain, peripheral edema, or palpitations, the prospect of valvular abnormalities, specifically tricuspid regurgitation, should be investigated with echocardiography. Tricuspid regurgitation is more prevalent in sickle cell disease and is associated with increased mortality [33–36].

10.9.3 Eye Complications

Eye complications in sickle cell disease in the form of proliferative sickle retinopathy and vitreous hemorrhage occur in 50% of patients and can result in significant vision loss. In proliferative sickle retinopathy, ischemia in eye vessels leads to neovascularization which, like diabetic retinopathy, leads to loss of vision. Laser photocoagulation therapy performed by an ophthalmologist is very helpful. Vitreous hemorrhages are a more severe complication of proliferative sickle retinopathy and in some cases may require surgical vitrectomy [29].

10.9.4 Priapism

Priapism, the occurrence of painful erections lasting over 4 hours, occurs in over a third of male patients with sickle cell disease, and most have their first occurrence before the age of 20 years [37]. For a number of reasons, a much lower percentage goes to the hospital for the treatment of sickle cell-related priapism [38]. Associated conditions that predispose a sickle cell patient to priapism are fever, asplenia, sexual arousal, and dehydration [38].

10.9.5 Stroke

Stroke, usually ischemic, occurs in up to 10% of children with sickle cell anemia and can cause weakness in the limbs, slurred speech, seizures, coma, and cognitive impairment. Recurrent strokes occur in a half to two thirds of untreated patients [39]. "Silent" cerebral infarctions are a particular problem that often go unnoticed but can cause significant neurological damage and cognitive disability. There are estimates that these silent stokes are present in up to a third of children with sickle cell disease and represent the most common neurological complication [39]. The presence of these silent strokes is usually detected on magnetic resonance imaging (MRI) and may be prompted by poor academic performance, increasing cognitive deficits, or falling intelligence quotients (IQ). The specific stroke trigger within a sickle cell patient population points to worsening anemia as a common cause. The anemia leads to increased cerebral demand for oxygen, and a cascade ending with infarction is the result. Given this rationale, transfusions are frequently the treatment for new strokes in sickle cell patients, and long-term repeated transfusions have been shown to be marginally effective in preventing recurrent strokes [40, 41].

10.9.6 Aplastic Crisis

Sickle cell patients presenting with sudden pallor and weakness in conjunction with dropping hemoglobin levels are having an aplastic crisis. The usual trigger is parvovirus B19 infection that suppresses the bone marrow's production of RBCs. This suppression of the bone marrow in combination with existing baseline anemia results in a very serious clinical state. Thankfully, the infection is self-limited, typically lasting 7–10 days [42].

10.9.7 Acute Chest Syndrome

Acute chest syndrome—ischemia and hypoxia due to vaso-occlusion of the pulmonary microvasculature—is the leading cause of death in patients with sickle cell disease [43]. It should be noted that as infection is the leading trigger of acute chest syndrome in children and adolescence, bone marrow or fat embolism is the leading trigger in adults. This is the most probable reason why this syndrome may have a more severe course and a higher mortality rate in adults [43]. Approximately 50% of patients with sickle cell will have an episode of acute chest syndrome in their lifetime. Although chest pain is the most frequent presenting symptom, this syndrome is frequently preceded or accompanied by vaso-occlusive pain crisis.

Acute chest syndrome is clinically defined as radiological evidence of a new pulmonary infiltrate, associated with one or more physical signs such as fever, chest pain, cough, tachypnea, or other signs of respiratory distress, including wheezing, rales, or hypoxia. Treatment goals involve managing the pain, alleviating the precipitating event (infection, dehydration, etc.) and anticipating and minimizing adverse sequelae. Emergent treatment includes intravenous fluid hydration, prophylactic antibiotics to address common organisms (*Mycoplasma*, *Chlamydia*, pneumococcus, *Haemophilus influenzae*), supplemental oxygen, and incentive spirometry. Simple or exchange transfusion can also be considered in moderate to severe acute chest syndrome. Patients with acute chest syndrome should also receive venous thromboembolism prophylaxis. Both hydroxyurea and chronic transfusion has been shown to reduce frequency of attacks [29]. Acute chest syndrome occurs with increased frequency in patients with a history of asthma or prior admission(s) for acute chest syndrome in the past [29].

10.9.8 Vaso-occlusive Pain Management

Pain is the most common reason patients with sickle cell disease seek medical attention. However, studies have shown healthcare providers tend to have a negative perception of an African American in pain that often interferes with conducting an adequate assessment and providing appropriate treatment [44–46]. The issues with the treatment of pain has worsened due to opioid restrictions imposed to address opioid abuse and overdose, yet the prevalence of opioid use disorders in patients with sickle cell is similar or lower than the general population [47]:

> with the exception of heart disease, the number of deaths due to opioid pain relievers in patients with sickle cell disease was less than other non-cancer pain conditions including fibromyalgia, low back pain, and migraine. Furthermore, the number of patients with sickle cell disease who died due to opioid pain relievers was significantly less than the total number of all patients with other diagnoses who died due to opioid pain relievers. [47]

The goal standard of pain assessment is self-reporting, as other clinical parameters and laboratory tests do not correlate with pain severity [48].

Patients with sickle cell become well aware of their triggers of pain and can usually predict or identify their precipitating event (infection, dehydration, cold, stressful events) [47, 49]. A recent study looked at and confirmed that stress can act as a trigger for vaso-occlusive crises:

> Baseline anxiety had a significant effect on the vasoconstriction response in sickle cell subjects but not controls. In conclusion, mental stress causes vasoconstriction and autonomic nervous system reactivity in all subjects. Although the pattern of responses were not

significantly different between two groups, the consequences of vasoconstriction can be quite significant in sickle cell disease because of the resultant entrapment of sickle cells in the microvasculature. This suggests that mental stress precipitates vaso-occlusive crisis in sickle cell disease by causing neural mediated vasoconstriction. [49]

It is important for healthcare professionals to be familiar with possible triggers and to encourage patients to be aware as well, as this may reduce painful episodes. Chronic pain management should be individualized, which encourages self-management of pain and adequate step-up therapy with the inclusion of opioids [48]. Hydroxyurea has also been shown to reduce pain episodes [50, 51]:

Although findings from the study of hydroxyurea in sickle cell disease indicate its beneficial effects in shortening the duration of crisis-related admissions and reducing the net dose of opioids, there have been concerns about its safety profile in pediatric sickle cell patients. Nevertheless, there is compelling evidence to support its use in patients as young as 9 months, given its reported ability to reduce the frequency of vaso-occlusive crises and acute chest syndrome with little or no adverse reactions. In fact, results from a protocol suggest minimal genotoxicity or carcinogenicity with long-term hydroxyurea exposure. A recent review further lends credence to its safety and efficacy in both pediatric and adult patients as there was no reported increase in the incidence of leukemia and teratogenicity. [50]

Patrick McGann and Russell Ware from Cincinnati Children's Hospital Medical Center rendered an expert opinion that "hydroxyurea therapy should be considered standard-of-care for (sickle cell anemia), representing an essential component of patient management. Early initiation and broader use of hydroxyurea will alter the natural history of (sickle cell anemia), so affected children can live longer and healthier lives" [51].

Acute painful episodes that require hospital visits need prompt and adequate analgesia. Opioids are usually the recommended medication and are to be given IV within 30 minutes of presentation. Rapid and frequent reassessment of pain is advised to achieve pain control, with adequate acceleration of dosage as indicated. Patient-controlled analgesia (PCA) pumps may also be indicated in patients with difficult to control pain. A slow and closely monitored tapered therapy of opioids to the patient's baseline should be encouraged as a part of discharge care planning [50].

10.10 Thalassemia (Alpha and Beta)

The thalassemias are a group of inherited autosomal recessive blood disorders that disproportionately affect African Americans by impairing hemoglobin production. Hemoglobin is the oxygen-transporting protein of red blood cells and has a quaternary structure consisting of four polypeptide subunits: two alpha chains and two beta chains. Alpha and beta thalassemias are hereditary disorders characterized by reductions in the synthesis of these chains, causing reduced successful hemoglobin production. The lower hemoglobin content reduces both the overall red blood cell production and the quality of individual red blood cells and results in hypochromic microcytic anemia [52].

Alpha thalassemia is caused by reduced or absent synthesis of alpha-globin chains, and beta thalassemia is caused by reduced or absent synthesis of beta-globin chains. Because of the quaternary structure, imbalances of the alpha- or beta-globin chains disrupt overall production.

Patients can be described as having the trait, intermedia, or major involvement. Patients with alpha or beta thalassemia trait are asymptomatic and require no treatment. Most persons with thalassemia trait are found incidentally when their blood count shows mild microcytic anemia. Another common classification separates transfusion dependent and non-transfusion dependent with African Americans comprising more non-transfusion-dependent patients [53].

In the intermedia or major thalassemia, the imbalance in the alpha- or beta-globin chain ratio leads to ineffective erythropoiesis, hemolytic anemia, hypercoagulability, and increased intestinal iron reabsorption. The body is retaining iron for red blood cell production, but because of the genetic imbalance, it cannot successfully complete the task. Anemia ensues, requiring transfusions and causing the iron body load to continue to rise. Transfusion-dependent patients will develop iron overload and require chelation therapy to remove the excess iron.

Thalassemia Minor: Minimal or no anemia (hemoglobin 9 to 12 g/dL); microcytosis; elevated RBC count

Thalassemia Intermedia: Microcytic anemia with hemoglobin usually higher than 7 g/dL; growth failure; hepatosplenomegaly; hyperbilirubinemia; thalassemic facies (i.e., frontal bossing, mandibular malocclusion, prominent malar eminences due to extramedullary hematopoiesis) develop between the ages of 2 and 5 years

Thalassemia Major (Cooley Anemia): Severe anemia (hemoglobin 1–6 g/dL) usually during the first year of life; hepatosplenomegaly; growth failure

Thalassemia affects men and women equally. Alpha thalassemia occurs most often in persons of African and Southeast Asian descent, and beta thalassemia is most common in persons of Mediterranean, African, and Southeast Asian descent. Thalassemia trait affects 5–30% of persons in these ethnic groups [52].

Persons with beta thalassemia major are diagnosed during infancy. Pallor, irritability, growth retardation, abdominal swelling, and jaundice appear during the first years of life.

The complications that occur with beta thalassemia major or intermedia are related to overstimulation of the bone marrow, ineffective erythropoiesis, and iron overload from regular blood transfusions.

If you have a healthy African American male with mild anemia, microcytosis, and no other associated abnormalities, think of thalassemia trait as a potential cause.

10.11 Glucose-6-Phosphate Dehydrogenase Deficiency (G6PD)

Glucose-6-phosphate dehydrogenase (G6PD) protects red blood cells from oxidative stress and hemolysis. G6PD deficiency is an inherited defect that makes red blood cells more susceptible to hemolysis. G6PD deficiency has a disproportionate occurrence among certain ethnic groups with approximately 12 percent prevalence in African Americans [54, 55]. This disorder, which is X-linked, usually presents with an acute hemolytic crisis that occurred after exposure to certain triggers, for example, the medication primaquine (an antimalarial medication). Patients are advised to stay away from such medications, fava beans, and chemicals such as henna and naphthalene which are potential triggers. Affected individuals should also be aware that infections as well as poor control of diabetes (e.g., DKA) could be potential triggers.

John Thomas and colleagues found an association between G6PG deficiency and cardiovascular disease:

> Our study suggests 39.6% greater odds of identifying CVD (cardiovascular disease) in G6PD-deficient individuals. To our knowledge, ours is the largest study to show this association. Universal screening of G6PD status—already performed in U.S. military personnel—might prove useful in the general population, leading to earlier cardiovascular screening and therapeutic intervention in people with G6PD deficiency. [56]

Treatment is aimed at supportive therapy for the acute hemolytic episode and the avoidance of triggers [57].

Important Differences in Hematology Results and Hematological Diseases

- African Americans may have significantly lower values in WBC, neutrophil count, monocyte count, and platelets.
- African Americans may have significantly lower values in hemoglobin (HGB), hematocrit (HCT), mean corpuscular hemoglobin (MCH), and mean corpuscular hemoglobin concentration (MCHC).
- Benign ethnic neutropenia (defined as between 1.0×10^9 cell/Liter and 1.5×10^9 cell/Liter) has increased prevalence in African American patients.
- When considering the general electrolytes, there are no significant differences in sodium, potassium, chloride, calcium, phosphorus, or magnesium between African Americans and European Americans.
- African Americans may have lower TSH levels with a range of 0.37–3.46 mIU/L (compared to "overall" reference interval 0.512–5.22 mIU/L).
- The lipid profile in African Americans is generally more favorable with a higher HDL and lower total cholesterol, LDL, and triglycerides.
- The prostate-specific antigen (PSA) test is a better and more sensitive detector of prostate cancer in African Americans, and at any given PSA level are at a higher risk for prostate cancer than European Americans.
- Significant differences in serum vitamin levels exist across the population with lower levels of vitamin D, vitamin B6, vitamin E, and folate. African Americans tend to have higher vitamin C and B12 levels.
- Sickle cell anemia occurs in 1 in 365 African American births. Sickle cell trait affects 1 in 13 African Americans.
- Annual screening and treatment with angiotensin-converting enzyme (ACE) inhibitors may delay renal disease progression in sickle cell disease.
- The spectrum of sickle hemoglobin-related nephropathy extends to sickle cell trait, with sickle cell trait conferring a twofold increased risk of chronic kidney disease.
- If African Americans with sickle cell disease have signs or symptoms suggestive of pulmonary hypertension, they should have echocardiography done (with particular attention to tricuspid regurgitation).
- End-stage renal disease is a rare complication but is associated with high mortality in sickle cell disease.
- Vision screening and ophthalmology evaluations should start early in sickle cell disease.

- Eye complications in sickle cell disease in the form of proliferative sickle retinopathy and vitreous hemorrhage occur in 50% of patients and can result in significant vision loss.
- Priapism is common affecting 35% of boys and men with sickle cell disease.
- Acute chest syndrome—ischemia and hypoxia due to vaso-occlusion of the pulmonary microvasculature—is the leading cause of death in patients with sickle cell disease.
- Thalassemia is a hereditary disorder characterized by reduction in synthesis of globin chains (α or β), causing reduced hemoglobin synthesis and eventually hypochromic microcytic anemia.
- Thalassemia has microcytosis out of proportion to the degree of anemia.
- Thalassemia has abnormal RBC morphology with microcytes, hypochromia, acanthocytes, and target cells.
- Thalassemias are described as:
  - *Trait*, when there are laboratory features without clinical impact.
  - *Intermedia*, when there is a RBC transfusion requirement or other moderate clinical impacts.
  - *Major*, when the disorder is life-threatening.
- G6PD deficiency has a disproportionate occurrence with approximately 12% prevalence in African Americans.

References

1. Harris K, Boyd JC. On dividing reference data into subgroups to produce separate reference ranges. Clin Chem. 1990;36/2:265–70.
2. Mayo Clinic, Author. Medical Laboratory Sciences. 2015. [June 15, 2015]. http://www.mayo.edu/mshs/careers/laboratory-sciences.
3. Hickner J, Thompson PJ, Wilkinson T, et al. Primary care physicians' challenges in ordering clinical laboratory tests and interpreting results. J Am Board Fam Med. 2014;27(2):268–74.
4. Lim E, Miyamura J, Chen JJ. Racial/ethnic-specific reference intervals for common laboratory tests: a comparison among Asians, Blacks, Hispanics, and White. Hawaii J Med Public Health. 2015;74(9):302–10.
5. Bain BJ. Ethnic and sex differences in the total and differential white cell count and platelet count. J Clin Pathol. 1996;49(8):664–6.
6. Hsieh MM, Everhart JE, Byrd-Holt DD, et al. Prevalence of neutropenia in the U.S. population: age, sex, smoking status, and ethnic differences. Ann Intern Med. 2007;146(7):486–92.
7. Reed WW, Diehl LF. Leukopenia, neutropenia, and reduced hemoglobin levels in healthy American blacks. Arch Intern Med. 1991;151:501–5.

8. Freedman DS, Gates L, Flanders WD, et al. Black/white differences in leukocyte subpopulations in men. Int J Epidemiol. 1997;26:757–64.
9. Lim EM, Cembrowski G, Cembrowski M, Clarke G. Race-specific WBC and neutrophil count reference intervals. Int J Lab Hematol. 2010;32(6p2):590–7.
10. Palmblad J, Hoglund P. Ethnic benign neutropenia: a phenomenon finds an explanation. Pediatr Blood Cancer. 2018;65(12):e27361. https://doi.org/10.1002/pbc.27361.
11. Lakhotia R, Aggarwal A, Link ME, et al. Natural history of benign ethnic neutropenia in individuals of African ancestry. Blood Cells Mol Dis. 2019;77:12–6.
12. Denic S, Narchi H, Mekaini A, et al. Prevalence of neutropenia in children by nationality. BMC Hematol. 2016;16:15.
13. Thobakgale CF, Ndung'u T. Neutrophil counts in persons of African origin. Curr Opin Hematol. 2014;21:50–7.
14. Hershman D, Weinberg M, Rosner Z, et al. Ethnic neutropenia and treatment delay in African American women undergoing chemotherapy for early-stage breast cancer. J Natl Cancer Inst. 2003;95:1545–8.
15. Tahmasebi H, Trajcevski K, Higgins V, Adeli K. Influence of ethnicity on population reference values for biochemical markers. Crit Rev Clin Lab Sci. 2018;55(5):359–75. https://doi.org/10.1080/10408363.2018.1476455. Epub 2018 Jun 6.
16. CLSI. Defining, establishing, and verifying reference intervals in the clinical laboratory; approved guideline. 3rd ed. CLSI document EP28-A3c. Vol. 28, No. 30. Wayne: Clinical and Laboratory Standards Institute; 2008.
17. Boucai L, Hollowell JG, Surks MI. An approach for development of age-, gender-, and ethnicity-specific thyrotropin reference limits. Thyroid. 2011;21(1):5–11. https://doi.org/10.1089/thy.2010.0092. Epub 2010 Nov 8.
18. Bentley AR, Rotimi CN. Interethnic differences in serum lipids and implications for cardiometabolic disease risk in African ancestry populations. Glob Heart. 2017;12(2):141–50.
19. Tang P, Du W, Xie K, et al. Characteristics of baseline PSA and PSA velocity in young men without prostate cancer: racial differences. Prostate. 2012;72:173–80.
20. Saraiya M, Kottiri BJ, Leadbetter S, et al. Total and percent free prostate-specific antigen levels among U.S. men, 2001–2002. Cancer Epidemiol Biomark Prev. 2005;14:2178–82.
21. Giri VH, Egleston B, Ruth K, et al. Race, genetic West African ancestry, and prostate cancer prediction by PSA in prospectively screened high-risk men. Cancer Prev Res (Phila). 2009;2(3):244–50.
22. Kallingal GJ, Walker MR, Musser JE, et al. Impact of race in using PSA velocity to predict for prostate cancer. Mil Med. 2014;179(3):329–32.
23. D'Amico AV, Chen MH, Roehl KA, et al. Preoperative PSA velocity and the risk of death from prostate cancer after radical prostatectomy. N Engl J Med. 2004;351:125–35.
24. Libon F, Cavalier E, Nikkels AF. Skin color is relevant to vitamin D synthesis. Dermatology (Basel). 2013;227:250–4.
25. Nessvi S, Johansson L, Jopson J, et al. Association of 25-hydroxyvitamin D3 levels in adult New Zealanders with ethnicity, skin color and self-reported skin sensitivity to sun exposure. Photochem Photobiol. 2011;87:1173–8.
26. Gozdzik A, Barta JL, Wu H, et al. Low wintertime vitamin D levels in a sample of healthy young adults of diverse ancestry living in the Toronto area: associations with vitamin D intake and skin pigmentation. BMC Public Health. 2008;8:336.

27. Kant AK, Graubard BI. Race-ethnic, family income, and education differentials in nutritional and lipid biomarkers in US children and adolescents: NHANES 2003–2006. Am J Clin Nutr. 2012;96:601–12.
28. Carmel R. Ethnic and racial factors in cobalamin metabolism and its disorders. Semin Hematol. 1999;36:88–100.
29. Yawn BP, Buchanan GR, Afenyi-Annan AN, et al. Management of sickle cell disease: summary of the 2014 evidence-based report by expert panel members. JAMA. 2014;312(10):1033–48.
30. Sickle Cell Disease|CDC. Retrieved from https://www.cdc.gov/ncbddd/sicklecell/facts.html.
31. Noronha SA, Sadremeli SC, Strouse JJ. Management of sickle cell disease in children. South Med J. 2016;109(9):495–502.
32. Naik RP, Derebail VK, Grams ME, et al. Association of sickle cell trait with chronic kidney disease and albuminuria in African Americans. JAMA. 2014;312:2115–25.
33. Naik RP, Derebail VK. The spectrum of sickle hemoglobin-related nephropathy: from sickle cell disease to sickle trait. Expert Rev Hematol. 2017;10(12):1087–94.
34. Fonseca GH, Salemi VC, Gualandro DM, Jardim C, Sousa R, Gualandro SF. Diagnosis of pulmonary hypertension in adults with sickle cell disease. Eur Heart J. 2010;31:759.
35. Liem RI, Nevin MA, Prestridge A, Young LT, Thompson AA. Tricuspid regurgitant jet velocity elevation and its relationship to lung function in pediatric sickle cell disease. Pediatr Pulmonol. 2009;44(3):281–9.
36. Arslankoylu AE, Hallioglu O, Yilgor E, Duzovali O. Assessment of cardiac functions in sickle cell anemia with Doppler myocardial performance index. J Trop Pediatr. 2010;56(3):195–7. https://www.cdc.gov/NCBDDD/sicklecell/data.html.
37. Adeyoju AB, Olujohungbe AB, Morris J, et al. Priapism in sickle-cell disease; incidence, risk factors and complications—an international multicentre study. BJU Int. 2002;90:898–902.
38. Dupervil B, Grosse S, Burnett A, Parker C. Emergency department visits and inpatient admissions associated with priapism among males with sickle cell disease in the United States, 2006–2010. PLoS One. 2016;11(4):e0153257.
39. Ohene-Frempong K, Weiner SJ, Sleeper LA, Miller ST, Embury S, Moohr JW, et al. Cerebrovascular accidents in sickle cell disease: rates and risk factors. Blood. 1998;91(1):288–94.
40. Fortin PM, Hopewell S, Estcourt LJ. Red blood cell transfusion to treat or prevent complications in sickle cell disease: an overview of cochrane reviews. Cochrane Database Syst Rev. 2018;(8):CD012082.
41. Estcourt LJ, Fortin PM, Hopewell S, et al. Blood transfusion for preventing primary and secondary stroke in people with sickle cell disease. Cochrane Database Syst Rev. 2013;(11):CD003146.
42. Hankins JS, Penkert RR, Lavoie P, et al. Original research: parvovirus B19 infection in children with sickle cell disease in the hydroxyurea era. Exp Biol Med (Maywood). 2016;241(7):749–54.
43. Dastgiri S, Dolatkhah R. Blood transfusions for treating acute chest syndrome in people with sickle cell disease. Cochrane Database Syst Rev. 2016;(8):CD007843. https://doi.org/10.1002/14651858.CD007843.pub3.
44. Haywood C, Diener-West M, Strouse J, et al. Perceived discrimination in health care is associated with a greater burden of pain in sickle cell disease. J Pain Symptom Manag. 2014;48(5):934–43.

45. Green CR, Anderson KO, Baker TA, et al. The unequal burden of pain: confronting racial and ethnic disparities in pain. Pain Med. 2003;4:277–94.
46. Burgess DJ, Grill J, Noorbaloochi S, et al. The effect of perceived racial discrimination on bodily pain among older African American men. Pain Med. 2009;10:1341–52.
47. Ruta NS, Ballas SK. The opioid drug epidemic and sickle cell disease: guilt by association. Pain Med. 2016;17(10):1793–8.
48. Chou R, Fanciullo GJ, Fine PG, et al. Clinical guidelines for the use of chronic opioid therapy in chronic noncancer pain. J Pain. 2009;10(2):113–30.
49. Shah P, Khaleel M, Thuptimdang W, et al. Mental stress causes vasoconstriction in sickle cell disease and normal controls. Haematologica. 2019. Pii: haematol 2018.211391.
50. Uwaezuoke SN, Ayuk AC, Ndu IK, et al. Vaso-occlusive crisis in sickle cell disease: current paradigm on pain management. J Pain Res. 2018;11:3141–50.
51. McGann PT, Ware RE. Hydroxyurea therapy for sickle cell anemia. Expert Opin Drug Saf. 2015;14(11):1749–58.
52. Muncie HL, Campbell J. Alpha and beta thalassemia. Am Fam Physician. 2009;80(4):339–44.
53. Vichinsky E, Cohen A, Thompson AA, et al. Epidemiologic and clinical characteristics of nontransfusion-dependent thalassemia in the United States. Pediatr Blood Cancer. 2018;65(7):e27067. https://doi.org/10.1002/pbc.27067. Epub 2018 Apr 10.
54. Nkhoma ET, Poole C, Vannappagari V, et al. The global prevalence of glucose-6-phosphate dehydrogenase deficiency: a systematic review and meta-analysis. Blood Cells Mol Dis. 2009;42:267–78.
55. Chinevere TD, Murry CK, Grant E, et al. Prevalence of glucose-6-phosphate dehydrogenase deficiency in U.S. Army personnel. Mil Med. 2006;17(9):905–7.
56. Thomas JE, Kang S, Wyatt CJ, et al. Glucose-6-phosphate dehydrogenase deficiency is associated with cardiovascular disease in U.S. military centers. Tex Heart Inst J. 2018;45(3):144–50.
57. Belfield KD, Tichy EM. Review and drug therapy implications of glucose-6-phosphate dehydrogenase deficiency. Am J Health Syst Pharm. 2018;75(3):97–104.

Important Differences in Gastroenterology

11

11.1 Hepatitis B

African Americans have the highest rate of acute hepatitis B infections of all racial groups in the United States with a two- to threefold higher prevalence of chronic hepatitis B infection [1]. Chronic hepatitis B is frequently asymptomatic, but long-term infection can lead to cirrhosis and/or hepatocellular carcinoma. Since the initiation of universal vaccination of newborn babies and catch-up vaccination of children and adolescents began in 1991, a steady and dramatic decline in hepatitis B infections has continued [2].

The principal modes of hepatitis B transmission across all US populations include IV drug users, the incarcerated/institutionalized, healthcare personnel, those needing multiple transfusions, organ transplant patients, those with multiple sex partners, and newborns to mothers with hepatitis B [3].

Hepatitis B infections are common among patients and staff of hemodialysis units. Up to half of the renal dialysis patients who contract hepatitis B become chronic carriers of the hepatitis B antigen allowing for multiple exposures to dialysis staff, transportation personnel, and close family contacts. The hepatitis B virus can remain viable on environmental surfaces for a week [4].

Kimberly Forde at the University of Pennsylvania reviewed ethnic disparities in chronic hepatitis B infections and reported the following [5]:

> Though there has been a decline in infection rates for all racial and ethnic groups from 2000–2014, African Americans continue to have the highest rate of new infections. New infections among African Americans were most often reported in patients who were male, 30–39 years of age, and those who engaged in high-risk behaviors that increase risk of transmission of hepatitis B infection, particularly use of intravenous (IV) drugs, men who have sex with men (MSM), and having two or more sexual partners. [5]

© Springer Nature Switzerland AG 2020

G. L. Hall, *Patient-Centered Clinical Care for African Americans*,

https://doi.org/10.1007/978-3-030-26418-5_11

Some of the persisting amplified risk in African Americans is the increased occurrence of hepatitis B and other sexually transmitted diseases (STD) in incarcerated and previously incarcerated African Americans. Information regarding exact numbers of infections in this population has been elusive but most report twice the occurrence [6] of hepatitis B and other STDs when compared to never incarcerated. It has been well established that African Americans compose a startling and disproportionate percentage of the incarcerated with the most recent percentage nationally of 37% compared to a 13% US population [7]. The increased incidence in this population leads to excess exposure to the communities in which they reside after release [8]:

> The most recent report of the burden of infectious diseases among prisoners and recently released individuals in the USA was presented to the Congress with data accurate to 1996, indicating disproportionately higher prevalence of chronic infections among these individuals than the general US population: HIV (nine-fold higher), AIDS (six-fold), HCV (ten-fold), HBV (five-fold), and tuberculosis (four-fold). [8]

Thirty percent of people reporting an acute hepatitis B infection have been incarcerated at some point prior [6, 8]. In addition, repeated incarcerations increase the risk for hepatitis B directly [6]. The highest prevalence of chronic hepatitis B was in HIV-positive populations [6].

In terms of testing and treatment for hepatitis B patients without immunity from vaccination, recent analysis by Hu et al. at the National Center for HIV, Viral Hepatitis, STDs, and TB Prevention looked at data for US ethnic minorities and found "more than half of racial/ethnic minority persons in these communities had not been tested for hepatitis B, and only about one-half of those who tested positive had ever received treatment" [9].

The major goal of hepatitis B therapy is to prevent the development of cirrhosis/liver failure and/or prevent hepatocellular carcinoma and its sequelae. Evidence of its benefit is presumed due to lower viral DNA [10]. Because the time it takes to progress from active infection to chronic infection to end-stage event takes many years, tracking this population over decades can be challenging.

Finally, the clinical course and consequences of hepatitis B infection are influenced by several factors including viral load, host immune status, environment, and viral genotypes (A–H). Different HBV genotypes are associated with different regions in the world [11, 12].

> Genotype A is widespread in sub-Saharan Africa, Northern Europe, and Western Africa; genotypes B and C are common in Asia; genotype C is primarily observed in Southeast Asia; genotype D is dominant in Africa, Europe, Mediterranean countries, and India; genotype G is reported in France, Germany, and the United States; and genotype H is commonly encountered in Central and South America. [11]

HBV genotypes are closely related with optimal treatment strategies for chronic hepatitis B patients. Genotype A HBV, which is more prevalent in people of sub-Saharan African descent, is associated with a more chronic and long-standing infection. Genotype A is also more responsive to accepted treatments like interferon-based therapy [11]. Unfortunately, this more indolent and long-term presence is also associated with a four- to fivefold increased risk for hepatocellular carcinoma [5]. Screen your older African Americans for hepatitis B, and then refer them for risk stratification and treatment.

11.2   Hepatitis C

African Americans are disproportionately infected by hepatitis C and represent 25% of the estimated 3.2 million people in the United States who are believed to be infected [13]. Younger African Americans are 1.6 times more likely to be chronically infected, and those over age 60 are 10 times more likely to have the infection [13]. These rates are likely underestimated as hepatitis prevalence studies often exclude vulnerable populations including African Americans [14]. It is also well established that African Americans have a lower response rate to current treatments [15]. Increased prevalence coupled with lower response to treatment makes for a dismal outlook, but there are interventions that clinicians can make that will have a very positive impact.

Overall, hepatitis C virus (HCV) infections are the leading cause of cirrhosis and hepatocellular carcinoma and the most common cause for liver transplantation [16]. Before the more widespread availability of newer direct-acting antiviral agents that "cure" hepatitis C, many African Americans were considered ineligible for treatment with interferon-based medications due to comorbidity contraindications that included seizures, cardiac diseases, hemoglobinopathies (sickle cell, thalassemia, etc.), bipolar disorder, and depression [17, 18].

Screen for Hepatitis C
- Current or prior IV drug users
- Transfusions prior to 1987
- Hemodialysis patients
- Persistently high ALT (alanine aminotransferase) levels
- HIV infection
- Organ transplant before 1992
- Blood exposure to someone with hepatitis C
- Children born to mothers with hepatitis C
- Patients with unlicensed or noncommercially obtained tattoos
- History of homelessness or incarceration

Aside from comorbidities that are contraindications to treatment with interferon-based therapies, African Americans disproportionately get infected with a hepatitis C virus with a genotype (currently there are 6 major genotypes and more than 50 subtypes) that is more difficult to treat. When these viral genotypes are examined by race, African Americans tended to have the more resistant strains [16].

The economic burden of hepatitis C extends deeply into hospitalization costs. Teshale, Xing, and colleagues at the Division of Viral Hepatitis at the Centers for Disease Control and Prevention found that African Americans had substantially higher hospital admission rates and length of stay [19].

Similar to other health conditions, despite the higher occurrence, African Americans tend to be screened less often for hepatitis C than European Americans and once diagnosed are referred for specialty care less often [20]. Stacey Trooskin and colleagues at Thomas Jefferson University discussed this curious disparity:

> Overall, minorities were less likely to be tested for HCV than whites in the presence of a known risk factor… The reason for low rates of testing among minorities in the presence of a risk factor is likely to be multifactorial. Practitioners may be more likely to ask minority patients about risk behaviors, given an implicit understanding of the surrounding urban community and the epidemiology of HCV, but less likely to test if the provider feels that the patient would not be a candidate for treatment or if the patient would not opt for treatment. [20]

This study also showed a significant referral bias against minorities. While 71% of European Americans with hepatitis C were referred for specialty care, only 32% of African Americans had evidence of a referral [20]. In contrast, studies have also shown that African Americans are more prone to decline interferon-based therapy after discussion with a specialist [21, 22]. Between lower referral rates and decreased acceptance on the patient's part, hepatitis C has been woefully addressed in African Americans.

Spontaneous clearance of hepatitis C occurs in up to half of acute infections overall, but studies involving African Americans show a much lower clearance incidence of closer to 10% [23, 24]. Researchers suspect that the overall higher prevalence in African Americans may be due to the lower clearance after the acute infection.

Despite the increased occurrence and lower clearance of hepatitis C in African Americans, there is a curious decrease in fibrosis and piecemeal necrosis of the liver [25]. Researchers suggest that the progression of hepatitis C may be slower in African Americans. This slower progression manifests itself as less hepatic necrosis, less liver fibrosis, and lower liver function tests, particularly ALT levels when compared to European American patients [26].

Direct-acting antiviral agents (DAAs) for hepatitis C are much more efficacious and have improved tolerability in all populations including African Americans; however, getting access to these medications has shown a significant disparity. Julia Marcus and colleagues looked at the initiation of these medications among Kaiser Permanente members (all insured) and found that racial/ethnic minorities (and persons of lower socioeconomic status) were much less likely to be prescribed these curative medicines [27]. They also found that reporting drug abuse, alcohol use, and/or smoking was also associated with a lower likelihood of being prescribed direct-acting antiviral agents. Omar Sims and researchers at the University of Alabama found a similar trend [28]:

Though DAAs have eliminated many historically, long-standing medical barriers to HCV treatment, several racial, psychological and socioeconomic barriers, and disparities remain. Consequently, patients who are African American, uninsured, and actively use drugs and alcohol will suffer from increased HCV-related morbidity and mortality in the coming years if deliberate public health and clinical efforts are not made to facilitate access to DAAs. [28]

While there are a number of challenges with African Americans and hepatitis C, thanks to newer medications, the future is bright. As clinicians properly profile, screen, and treat African Americans with hepatitis C, the overall burden of this disease will fade. Kendall Beck and colleagues at the University of California confirmed that [29]:

despite the known medical and psychosocial challenges faced by underserved (African American) populations, the availability of DAA-based therapies has significantly improved treatment eligibility, treatment initiation, treatment success, as well as adherence to HCV care compared to pre-DAA era therapies. DAA access appears to be the single most important factor influencing engagement with HCV care among the underserved African American population. Thus, eliminating the barrier of access to DAA regimens will likely significantly reduce hepatitis C disparities, a public health priority, in this underserved population. [29]

11.3 Hepatocellular Carcinoma

Because hepatocellular carcinoma (HCC) is so frequently a result of long-standing hepatitis B and C infection in African Americans, it is better reviewed in close conjunction with these infections (rather than in Chap. 6). African Americans have an increased risk for hepatocellular carcinoma and the related mortality [30]. Yu and colleagues at the University of Maryland looked at the incidence of hepatocellular carcinoma and found dramatically increased rate in African Americans and the patients were "much younger" than European American patients [31]. They noted a median age with HCC of 53 in African Americans compared to 67 in European Americans. They also found an increased occurrence of hepatitis B, hepatitis C, co-occurring hepatitis B and C, and hepatitis B and C with diabetes. Finally, there was a twofold decreased occurrence of alcoholic liver disease in African Americans [31].

Hepatitis C is the most common risk factor for hepatocellular carcinoma and is found in 25% of cases. The hepatitis C cases were also associated with younger age and therefore earlier infection. Concurrent hepatitis B and C infections increased the risk for hepatocellular carcinoma by 2–20 times compared with hepatitis B alone, and alcoholic liver disease plus hepatitis C was associated with a 200–400% increase risk compared with hepatitis C alone.

Diabetes increased the relative risk of hepatocellular carcinoma by 60–500% in individuals with hepatitis B, hepatitis C, and alcoholic liver disease. Hepatitis B and C were twice as prevalent among African American than European American patients, and those two infections comprised half of the hepatocellular carcinomas in African American patients [31].

Like other cancers, early detection is the key to improved prognosis in hepatocellular carcinoma. Amy Kim and Amit Singal looked at health disparities in the early detection of hepatocellular carcinoma [30]:

> Guidelines from the American Association for the Study of Liver Diseases (AASLD) recommend HCC surveillance in patients with cirrhosis and/or chronic HBV using ultrasound every 6 months. Surveillance is efficacious for early stage detection and is associated with higher rates of curative treatment and improved survival in at-risk patients. However, despite a strong evidence base and guideline recommendations, less than 20% of patients with cirrhosis currently receive surveillance. Underuse of surveillance may be mediated by patient-level factors (e.g. non-adherence), provider-level factors (e.g. lack of knowledge or disbelief regarding benefits of HCC surveillance), and/or system-level factors (e.g. lack of access to medical care). [30]

In the Surveillance Epidemiology and End Results (SEER)-Medicare database, African Americans had the lowest screening rate for hepatocellular carcinoma at 12%, European Americans were 15%, Hispanic/Latino were 17%, and Asian Americans had the highest screening rate at 28%. Overall, patients with the higher median income and/or educational levels were more likely to be screened [32].

Once detected, the prognosis for hepatocellular carcinoma depends on the tumor stage at diagnosis. Early detection of hepatocellular carcinoma and treatment with resection, ablation, or transplantation can result in a 5-year survival rate of over 70% [33]. Unfortunately, African Americans are less likely to be referred for resection, ablation, or liver transplantation [33].

11.4   Inflammatory Bowel Diseases

Inflammatory bowel diseases are conventionally believed to occur disproportionately more in European Americans, but their occurrence is progressing in other minorities including African Americans. Satimai Aniwan and colleagues at the Mayo Clinic looked at the incidence and trends over 40 years. They found a 134% increase in occurrence in minorities from 1970 to 2010 [34]. With this progression, the incidence is still much lower in African Americans and is estimated at two thirds the rate of European Americans.

11.4.1 Crohn's Disease and Ulcerative Colitis

Crohn's disease may involve any part of the gastrointestinal tract and is often associated with extraintestinal manifestations, perianal disease, strictures, and fistulas [35]. Studies have suggested that African Americans tend to have more perianal disease, uveitis, and sacroiliitis compared to European Americans [36] but other larger studies have failed to confirm this finding [37]. Cigarette smoking is strongly associated with the development of this disease, and continued smoking is associated with recurrence and worse outcomes. A study by Sofia, Rubin, and colleagues found that African Americans had more prominent joint symptoms linked with Crohn's disease activity [38].

A racial disparity in specialty referrals, emergency department use, and higher-end medical therapies was found in patients with Crohn's and ulcerative colitis by Geoffrey Nguyen and colleagues at John Hopkins University [39]:

> our study provides additional evidence of racial disparities in the field of IBD (inflammatory bowel disease) that may impact the overall effectiveness of medical therapy. Clinical trials tout the potent efficacy of biologics, but these results were derived under ideal study conditions, in which minorities are underrepresented. The relatively lower utilization of specialist care and anti-TNF agents among (African Americans) outside of a protocol-driven milieu may generate racial differences in how well the efficacy of clinical trials is translated into real-world effectiveness. [39]

Surgical interventions were reviewed by Eliot Arsoniadis and colleagues at the University of Minnesota and found that African Americans had a greater number of postoperative complications [40].

11.5 GERD

Gastroesophageal reflux disease (GERD) has a similar (and common) occurrence in African Americans when compared to European Americans but has a much lower transformation to endoscopy-confirmed esophagitis or adenocarcinoma [41, 42]. El-Serag and colleagues from Baylor College of Medicine make the following observation:

> Our findings indicate that (African Americans) and (European Americans) in the United States have a similar prevalence of GERD symptoms. Remarkably, (African Americans) have a lower prevalence of esophagitis than (European Americans) for the same frequency and severity of GERD symptoms. Irrespective of race, monthly GERD symptoms were present in more than one half and weekly symptoms were present in approximately one fourth of all participants. [41]

Esophageal adenocarcinoma has a fourfold increased rate in European Americans with similar prevalence of GERD across populations [41].

11.6 Barrett's Esophagus

While gastroesophageal reflux disease prevalence seems to be the same across races, Barrett's esophagus also has a curiously decreased prevalence in African Americans [43]. Ahmad Alkaddour and colleagues at the University of Florida looked at over 15,000 endoscopies and found a confirmed decreased occurrence of mucosal changes consistent with Barrett's esophagus in African Americans [43]. This decreased occurrence was despite similarities in GERD history, cigarette/alcohol use, medications prescribed, and body mass index. There is also a decreased risk for Barrett's esophagus following erosive esophagitis formation in African Americans [44].

11.7 *Helicobacter pylori*

The overall prevalence of *Helicobacter pylori* infections in the United States has declined over the past 60 years as the availability of antibiotics and acid blockers has increased [45, 46]. Unfortunately, the prevalence has not declined in African Americans as distinctly as in European Americans [45]. Theresa Nguyen and colleagues looked at the prevalence of *H. pylori* in 1200 veterans in Texas and found over half of the African American men were positive for *H. pylori* compared to under 10% of European Americans [47]. Some of the increased *H. pylori* risk was related to socioeconomic factors, but these did not account for all of the differences [47].

11.8   Gallbladder Disease

Despite the higher risk of gallbladder disease with increasing obesity rates, there is a slightly decreased risk for gallstone formation and subsequent disease in African Americans [48, 49].

Sickle cell disease is associated with the formation of gallstones that frequently progress to cholecystitis. Because a sickle cell crisis may present with similar symptoms, prophylactic cholecystectomy should be strongly considered when stones are noted [49]. Complications from surgery, whether planned or emergent, are significant [49].

Important Differences in Gastroenterological Diseases
- African Americans have the highest rate of acute hepatitis B virus (HBV) infections of all racial groups in the United States with a two- to threefold higher prevalence.
- African Americans with a history of incarceration have a greatly increased risk for hepatitis B, hepatitis C, and other sexually transmitted diseases.
- HBV genotypes are closely related with optimal treatment strategies for chronic hepatitis B patients, and type A is most frequent in African Americans and more responsive to interferon-based therapy.
- While African Americans comprise approximately 13% of the US population, they make up approximately 25% of the hepatitis C population.
- African Americans disproportionately get infected with a hepatitis C virus with a genotype that is more difficult to treat.
- African Americans' clearance of hepatitis C after acute infection occurs at a much lower rate and accounts for some of the increased overall prevalence.
- Despite the increased occurrence and lower clearance of hepatitis C in African Americans, there is a curious decrease in fibrosis and piecemeal necrosis of the liver upon biopsy.
- Despite the higher occurrence of both hepatitis B and C, African Americans tend to be screened less often and once diagnosed are referred for specialty care less often.
- The availability of DAA-based therapies for HCV cure has significantly improved treatment eligibility, treatment initiation, and treatment successes in African American patients.

- African Americans have increased risk for hepatocellular carcinoma and the related mortality, and it occurs at a significantly earlier age (age 53 vs. 67 in European Americans).
- African Americans have the lowest screening rate for hepatocellular carcinoma despite the increased risk.
- Once diagnosed with HCC, African Americans are less likely to be referred for resection, ablation, or liver transplantation.
- Inflammatory bowel diseases occur disproportionately less often in African Americans.
- African Americans with Crohn's disease have more prominent joint symptoms and possibly more perianal disease.
- Stressing smoking cessation in patients with Crohn's disease is critical.
- African Americans requiring surgery for Crohn's disease have a greater number of postoperative complications.
- GERD has a similar occurrence in African Americans when compared to European Americans but has a much lower transformation to esophagitis or adenocarcinoma.
- Barrett's esophagus has a decreased prevalence in African Americans.
- There is a higher prevalence of *Helicobacter pylori* infections in African Americans.
- There is a marginally decreased risk for gallbladder disease in African Americans when compared to European Americans.
- Sickle cell disease is associated with the formation of gallstones that frequently progress to cholecystitis. Because a sickle cell crisis may present with similar symptoms, prophylactic cholecystectomy should be strongly considered when stones are noted.

References

1. Forde KA, Tanapanpanit O, Reddy KR. Hepatitis B and C in African Americans: current status and continued challenges. Clin Gastroenterol Hepatol. 2014;12(5):738–48.
2. Wasley A, Kruszon-Moran D, Kuhnert W, Simard EP, Finelli L, McQuillan G, et al. The prevalence of hepatitis B virus infection in the United States in the era of vaccination. J Infect Dis. 2010;202(2):192–201.
3. Carroll KC, Hobden JA, Miller S, Morse SA, Mietzner TA, Detrick B, Mitchell TG, McKerrow JH, Sakanari JA, editors. Hepatitis viruses. In: Jawetz, Melnick, & Adelberg's medical microbiology. New York: McGraw-Hill. p. 27e; http://0-accessmedicine.mhmedical.com.crusher.neomed.edu/content.aspx?bookid=1551&sectionid=94109875. Accessed 12 May 2019.

4. Hepatitis B Questions and Answers for the Public. Centers for Disease Control and Prevention. https://www.cdc.gov/hepatitis/hbv/bfaq.htm. Accessed 12 May 2019.
5. Forde F. Ethnic disparities in chronic hepatitis B infection: African American and Hispanic Americans. Curr Hepatol Rep. 2017;16(2):105–12.
6. Hennessey KA, Kim AA, Griffin V, et al. Prevalence of infection with hepatitis B and C viruses and co-infection with HIV in three jails: a case for viral hepatitis prevention in jails in the United States. J Urban Health. 2009;86(1):93–105.
7. Statistics Inmate Race. Federal Bureau of Prisons. 2019. https://www.bop.gov/about/statistics/statistics_inmate_race.jsp. Accessed 12 May 2019.
8. Gupta S, Altice FL. Hepatitis B virus infection in US correctional facilities: a review of diagnosis, management, and public health implications. J Urban Health. 2009;86(2):263–79.
9. Hu DJ, Xing J, Tohme RA, Liao Y, Pollack H, Ward JW, et al. Hepatitis B testing and access to care among racial and ethnic minorities in selected communities across the United States, 2009–2010. Hepatology. 2013;58(3):856–62.
10. Sorrell MF, Belongia EA, Costa J, et al. National institutes of health consensus development conference of hepatitis B. Ann Intern Med. 2009;150(2):104–10.
11. Sunbul M. Hepatitis B virus genotypes: global distribution and clinical importance. World J Gastroenterol. 2014;20(18):5427–34.
12. DiBisceglie AM, King WC, Lisker-Melman M, et al. Age, race and viral genotype are associated with the prevalence of hepatitis B antigen in children and adults with chronic hepatitis. J Viral Hepat. 2019. https://doi.org/10.1111/jvh.13104. Assessed 12 May 2019.
13. Denniston MM, Jiles RB, Drobeniuc J, et al. Hepatitis C virus infection in the United States, national health and nutrition examination survey 2003 to 2010. Ann Intern Med. 2014;160(5):293–300.
14. Wilder J, Saraswathula A, Hasselblad V, Muir A. A systematic review of race and ethnicity in hepatitis C clinical trial enrollment. J Natl Med Assoc. 2016;108(1):24–9.
15. Conjeevaram HS, Fried MW, Jeffers LJ, et al. Peginterferon and ribavirin treatment in African American and Caucasian American patients with hepatitis C genotype 1. Gastroenterology. 2006;131(2):470–7.
16. Saab S, Jackson C, Nieto J, Francois F. Hepatitis C in African Americans. Am J Gastroenterol. 2014;109(10):1576–84.
17. Talal AH, LaFleur J, Hoop R, et al. Absolute and relative contraindications to pegylated-interferon or ribavirin in the US general patient population with chronic hepatitis C: results from a US database of over 45 000 HCV-infected, evaluated patients. Aliment Pharmacol Ther. 2013;37(4):473–81.
18. Rowan PJ, Tabasi S, Abdul-Latif M, et al. Psychosocial factors are the most common contraindications for antiviral therapy at initial evaluation in veterans with chronic hepatitis C. J Clin Gastroenterol. 2004;38:530–4.
19. Teshale EH, Xing J, Moorman A, et al. Higher all-cause hospitalization among patients with chronic hepatitis C: the Chronic Hepatitis C Cohort Study (CHeCS), 2006–2013. J Viral Hepat. 2016;23(10):748–54.
20. Trooskin SB, Navarro VJ, Winn RJ, et al. Hepatitis C risk assessment, testing and referral for treatment in urban primary care: role of race ethnicity. World J Gastroenterol. 2007;13(7):1074–8.

21. Khokhar OS, Lewis JH. Reasons why patients infected with chronic hepatitis C virus choose to defer treatment: do they alter their decision with time? Dig Dis Sci. 2007;52(5):1168–76.
22. Borum ML, Igiehon E, Shafa S, et al. African Americans may differ in their reasons for declining hepatitis C therapy compared to non-African Americans. Dig Dis Sci. 2009;54:1604–5.
23. Thomas DL, Astemborski J, Rai RM, et al. The natural history of hepatitis c virus infection: host, viral, and environmental factors. JAMA. 2000;284:450–6.
24. Mir HM, Stepanova M, Afendy M, et al. African Americans are less likely to have clearance of hepatitis C virus infection: the findings from recent U.S. population data. J Clin Gastroenterol. 2012;46(8):e62–5.
25. Sterling RK, Stravitz RT, Luketic VA, et al. A comparison of the spectrum of chronic hepatitis C virus between Caucasians and African Americans. Clin Gastroenterol Hepatol. 2004;2(6):469–73.
26. Crosse K, Umeadi OG, Anania FA, et al. Racial difference in liver inflammation and fibrosis related to chronic hepatitis C. Clin Gastroenterol Hepatol. 2004;2(6):463–8.
27. Marcus JL, Hurley LB, Chamberland S. Disparities in initiation of direct-acting antiviral agents for hepatitis C virus infection in an insured population. Public Health Rep. 2018;133(4):452–60.
28. Sims OT, Guo Y, Shoreibah MG, et al. Short article: alcohol and substance use, race, and insurance status predict nontreatment for hepatitis C virus in the era of direct acting antivirals: a retrospective study in a large urban tertiary center. Eur J Gastroenterol Hepatol. 2017;29(11):12191222.
29. Beck KR, Kim NJ, Khalili M. Direct acting antivirals improve HCV treatment initiation and adherence among underserved African Americans. Ann Hepatol. 2018;17(3):413–8.
30. Kim AK, Singal AG. Health disparities in diagnosis and treatment of hepatocellular carcinoma. Clin Liver Dis (Hoboken). 2015;4(6):143–5.
31. Yu L, Sloane DA, Guo C, Howell CD. Risk factors for primary hepatocellular carcinoma in black and white Americans in 2000. Clin Gastroenterol Hepatol. 2006;4(3):355–60.
32. Davila JA, Morgan RO, Richardson PA, et al. Use of surveillance for hepatocellular carcinoma among patients with cirrhosis in the United States. Hepatology. 2010;52:132–41.
33. Zak Y, Rhoads KF, Visser BC. Predictors of surgical intervention for hepatocellular carcinoma: race, socioeconomic status, and hospital type. Arch Surg. 2011;146(7):778–84.
34. Aniwan S, Harmsen WS, Tremaine WJ, et al. Incidence of inflammatory bowel disease by race and ethnicity in a population-based inception cohort from 1970 through 2010. Ther Adv Gastroenterol. 2019;12:1756284819827692.
35. McQuaid KR. Gastrointestinal disorders. In: Papadakis MA, McPhee SJ, Rabow MW, editors. Current medical diagnosis & treatment. New York: McGraw-Hill; 2019; http://0-accessmedicine.mhmedical.com.crusher.neomed.edu/content.aspx?bookid=2449&sectionid=194439115. Accessed 05 June 2019.
36. Nguyen GC, Torres EA, Regueiro M, et al. Inflammatory bowel disease characteristics among African Americans, Hispanics, and non-Hispanic Whites: characterization of a large North American cohort. Am J Gastroenterol. 2006;101(5):1012–23.
37. Bertha M, Vasantharoopan A, Kumar A, et al. IBD Serology and disease outcomes in African Americans with Crohn's disease. Inflamm Bowel Dis. 2018;24(1):209–16.
38. Sofia MA, Rubin DT, Hou N, Pekow J. Clinical presentation and disease course of inflammatory bowel disease differs by race in a large tertiary care hospital. Dig Dis Sci. 2014;59(9):2228–35.

39. Nguyen GC, LaVeist TA, Harris ML, et al. Racial disparities in utilization of specialist care and medications in inflammatory bowel disease. Am J Gastroenterol. 2010;105(10):2202–8.

40. Arsoniadis EG, Ho YY, Melton GB, Madoff RD, et al. African Americans and short-term outcomes after surgery for Crohn's disease: an ACS-NSQIP analysis. J Crohns Colitis. 2017;11(4):468–73.

41. El-Serag HB, Petersen NJ, Carter J, et al. Gastroesophageal reflux among different racial groups in the United States. Gastroenterology. 2004;126(7):1692–9.

42. Spechler SJ, Jain SK, Tendler DA, Parker RA. Racial differences in the frequency of symptoms and complications of gastro-oesophageal reflux disease. Aliment Pharmacol Ther. 2002;16(10):1795–800.

43. Alkaddour A, McGaw C, Hritani R, et al. Protective propensity of race or environmental features in the development of Barrett's esophagus in African Americans – a single center pilot study. J Natl Med Assoc. 2019;111(2):198–201.

44. Alkaddour A, McGaw C, Hritani R, et al. African American ethnicity is not associated with development of Barrett's esophagus after erosive esophagitis. Dig Liver Dis. 2015;47(10):853–6.

45. Grad Y, Lipsitch M, Aiello AE. Secular trends in *Helicobacter pylori* seroprevalence in adults in the United States: evidence for sustained race/ethnic disparities. Am J Epidemiol. 2012;175(1):54–9.

46. Parsonnet J. The incidence of *Helicobacter pylori* infection. Aliment Pharmacol Ther. 1995;9(suppl 2):45–51.

47. Nguyen T, Ramsey D, Graham D, et al. The prevalence of *Helicobacter pylori* remains high in African Americans and Hispanic veterans. Helicobacter. 2015;20(4):305–15.

48. Stinton LM, Shaffer EA. Epidemiology of gallbladder disease: cholelithiasis and cancer. Gut Liver. 2012;6(2):172–87.

49. Figueiredo JC, Haiman C, Porcel J, et al. Sex and ethnic/racial-specific risk factors for gallbladder disease. BMC Gastroenterol. 2017;17(1):153.

Other Important Differences in Clinical Care

12

12.1 Pain

Ethnic differences in pain perception have been documented with most researchers agreeing that African Americans have greater pain sensitivity and lower pain tolerance. Edwards and colleagues at the University of Alabama confirmed that:

> African American subjects reported higher levels of clinical pain as well as greater pain-related disability than (European American) participants. In addition, substantial group differences were observed for ischemic pain tolerance, with African Americans demonstrating less tolerance than (European Americans). [1]

Campbell and colleagues at the College of Clinical and Health Psychology at the University of Florida examined racial/ethnic differences in response to a variety of experimental pain stimuli. They again found "African Americans had lower tolerances for a variety of pains including heat pain, cold pressor pain and ischemic pain" when compared to European Americans [2].

With the added burden of worse disease outcomes and premature death due to a myriad of health problems, it is no surprise that there is also a significant racial disparity in the treatment of pain [3]. Whether it is due to access issues and insurance, bias and discrimination in the healthcare system, or poor-quality communication with their providers, African Americans are more likely to have whatever pain they have go undertreated or untreated. Based on a number of studies, African Americans are more likely to have their pain discounted or underestimated and less likely to be screened for pain [4–7].

The unequal treatment of pain in African Americans spans their lifetime. A study of nearly one million children diagnosed with appendicitis revealed that,

© Springer Nature Switzerland AG 2020
G. L. Hall, *Patient-Centered Clinical Care for African Americans*,
https://doi.org/10.1007/978-3-030-26418-5_12

relative to European American children, African American children were less likely to receive any pain medication for moderate pain and were less likely to receive opioids for severe pain [8]. African American adults with identical joint surgeries had demonstrably decreased pain treatment. As Anderson and colleagues found in their study [7] "Racial and ethnic disparities in pain: causes and consequences of unequal care":

> This review reveals the persistence of racial and ethnic disparities in acute, chronic, cancer, and palliative pain care across the lifespan and treatment settings, with minorities receiving lesser quality pain care than (European Americans).

Another study involving medical record review of equal pain symptoms in racially matched patients found African Americans with lower rates of receiving pain medications, and the cause was ultimately attributed to physician discretion [4].

Meghani, Byun, and Gallagher at the University of Pennsylvania looked at 25 years of data regarding pain treatment and found [9]:

> Blacks/African Americans experienced both a higher number and magnitude of disparities than any other group in the analyses... In subanalyses, opioid treatment disparities for Blacks/African Americans remained consistent across pain types, settings, study quality, and data collection periods.

Many studies have documented decreased use of opioids in African Americans with disparities persisting to the present day [10–13]. One objective approach to determining opioid-prescribing disparities simply looked at a population of Medicaid beneficiaries in North Carolina with chronic non-cancer pain. Ringwalt and colleagues at the University of North Carolina at Chapel Hill looked at over 75,000 Medicaid patients with chronic non-cancer pain and simply tracked prescriptions filled for pain [11]. By cross-referencing prescriber specialty and self-reported race, they found that African Americans:

> ... were 9% less likely than (European Americans) to fill an opioid prescription, when controlling for age, sex, and chronic pain diagnosis. OB/GYN, internal medicine, and general practice/family medicine specialties were primary contributors to this disparity; relative to (European Americans) CNCP (chronic non-cancer pain) beneficiaries, (African American) CNCP beneficiaries were 22%, 14%, and 9% less likely to fill opioid prescriptions, respectively. [11]

By tracking prescription attainment data and controlling for ability to pay for the prescription (all were Medicaid), this large study again confirmed prescribing disparities based on race:

Of all prescriptions filled by (European American) and (African American) beneficiaries with CNCP (chronic non-cancer pain), 12.6% were for opioids... Every specialty, with the exception of ENT physicians, wrote a greater proportion of opioid prescriptions for (European Americans) than for (African Americans) ... we have not only replicated earlier findings regarding differential race-based opioid dispensing, but have also revealed the presence of differences in race-based dispensing by provider specialty." [11]

The verified decreased use of pain medications in a population with an objectively lower threshold for pain, and a protracted need due to increased comorbidities, is unusually ironic and incredibly cruel.

The recent opioid crisis has shown a distinct racial difference between European Americans and other racial minorities with regard to opioid-related intoxications, accidental death, and suicides. Feng, Iser, and Yang in a Nevada study of emergency care showed a consistent decreased occurrence of opioid-related abuse in minorities, including African Americans [12]:

Results from this study indicate that NHWs (European Americans) had greater opioid-related health service utilization than nonwhites. In light of previous evidence on similar racial disparities, this pattern may suggest that nonwhite individuals did not experience the pain reduction benefits or associated risks of opioid medications to the same degree as NHWs (European Americans). [12]

"At-Risk" Signs of Potential Opioid Abuse [12]
- Co-occurring psychiatric disorders (depression, bipolar, etc.)
- Past cocaine use or abuse
- Convictions for driving under the influence
- Past alcohol or drug problems
- Daily nicotine use
- Obesity
- Long-term use of benzodiazepines
- Long-term use of sleep aids including zolpidem, zaleplon, and eszopiclone

With the recent opioid crisis, it is completely appropriate to stratify the risk of addiction based on accepted clinical criteria no matter the race or ethnicity. African Americans can, and do, get addicted to pain medications; however, their historical undertreatment coupled with well-intentioned endeavors to curb opioid addiction and related accidental death could widen an already-gapping disparity for a population at lessor risk for abuse.

12.1.1 Better Understanding

Sometimes reactions and dynamics between providers and patient differ based purely on social strategies. For example, the Center for Chronic Disease Outcomes Research found that "challenging" or "angry" African American patients were more likely to have their opioid pain medication dosage increased, whereas the opposite or "non-challenging" behavior in European American patients leads to more likely increased dosages [13]:

> Results point to the need for better understanding of the way a complex interplay of non-clinical characteristics affects physician behavior in order to improve quality of pain management and other clinical decision-making. [13]

This study simply looked at what works when it comes to provider behavior ... and an aggressive African American was more likely to get an accommodation from a provider. Prior knowledge of this can help explain an irate African American patient's behavior and provide a perspective for knowing that the patient is only using a tried and true approach. Communicating with the patient in a non-confrontational way and one that puts the patient's best interest first will diffuse many unpleasant interactions. Continuing to review outcomes as it relates to African Americans should be the goal of providers with high African American populations. Provider ethnic literacy allows for a more fluid provision of care through better preparation and understanding.

In summary, African Americans have an increased sensitivity to all types of pain, particularly ischemic pain, are dramatically undertreated for their pain throughout their life, and have a comparatively lower risk for abuse and addiction. Always consider a patient's abuse potential, but also consider the pain and suffering that can be treated. Pain still exists in African Americans every day, err on the side of treating it.

12.2   Mental Illness

Overall, African Americans tend to have fewer mental illnesses when compared to European Americans with significantly less anxiety, depression, and suicide [14–19]. Across racial groups, women tend to have higher rates of diagnosed depression and anxiety disorders than men, but men have higher rates of diagnosed substance abuse and related suicide [14].

African American men are less likely to seek the help of a psychiatric professional than European American men, and their presentation can be different. Sidney Hankerson at Columbia University looked at treatment disparities among African American men and made the following observations:

Racial and gender differences in depressive symptomatology may contribute to the misdiagnosis of depression among African American men. The core symptoms of MDD (major depressive disorder) are remarkably consistent across cultures, however, African Americans with MDD are more likely to have somatic symptoms (e.g., sleep disturbance or pain) compared to (European) Americans with MDD. African Americans' somatization of emotional problems may make it difficult for primary care physicians to detect clinical depression. Researchers have increasingly studied a "male depressive syndrome" to describe how men experience and express depression. Depressed men, compared with women, are more likely to exhibit irritability, anger attacks, and abusive behavior. Men may be more likely to engage in externalizing behaviors, such as substance abuse and over-working, as a way to cope with depressive episodes. These gender differences in symptom presentation may lead to under-detection and misdiagnosis. [15]

Some of the "under-detection" of depression and other mood disorders is provider-driven and has its roots in bias. African Americans are disproportionately more diagnosed with schizophrenia and other psychotic disorders while less often diagnosed with mood disorders like depression and anxiety [15]. Cultural mistrust of medical providers is frequently attributed to paranoia rather than a variation in perspective [20]. Derek Suite and colleagues wrote about this phenomenon:

> … it may not be readily apparent to the treatment provider who interacts with a person of color that more than 200 years' worth of anecdotal and documentary evidence on racism in medicine and mental health cuts across age, gender and different racial/ethnic groups, leading to a high degree of vigilance, mistrust and disdain towards the medical establishment in general and mental health in particular. [21]

Arthur Whaley looked at the impact of gender- and race-matching patients and providers and found increased diagnostic accuracy when an African American male provider assessed an African American male patient with a strong racial identity [20]. The shared history (and reality) between race-matched providers and patients allowed for improved connections.

Researchers also noted that African Americans have higher stress levels than European Americans [19]. Having higher stress levels yet lower major depressive episodes forms the basis for another racial paradox:

> Major epidemiologic studies in the US reveal a consistent "paradox" by which psychiatric outcomes such as major depressive disorder (MDD) are less prevalent among (African Americans) relative to (European Americans), despite greater exposure to social and economic stressors and worse physical health outcomes. A second paradox, which has received less attention and has never been systematically documented, is the discrepancy between these patterns and (African American-European American) comparisons in psychological distress, which reveal consistently higher levels among (African Americans). [19]

The *Chartbook on Health Care for Blacks* published by the National Healthcare Quality and Disparities Report looked at quality measures related to depression and suicide and showed a narrowing disparity as both depression and suicide increase in African Americans. It also clearly demonstrated the decreased occurrence of depression and suicide [22] (Figs. 12.1 and 12.2).

As scholars try to understand why African Americans, with all of the increased disease and premature death, would have a lower psychiatric burden, an array of theories have been proposed. Keep in mind that these theories are merely hypotheses that have yet to be confirmed or refuted. Like anything in medicine, sometimes the best answer is "it is what it is" … just as African Americans bear an increased burden in the kidney and cardiovascular disease, they show an overall decreased burden psychiatrically. Since other theories were advanced for why other disease burdens exist, it is also fair to look at postulates here.

Jackson and colleagues at the University of Michigan proposed that increased stress leads to unhealthy coping mechanisms (like drug use) that protect against severe mental illness but adds to morbidity and premature mortality [16]:

Thus, we hypothesize that when individuals are chronically confronted with stressful conditions in daily life (e.g., poverty, crime, poor housing), they will engage in unhealthy

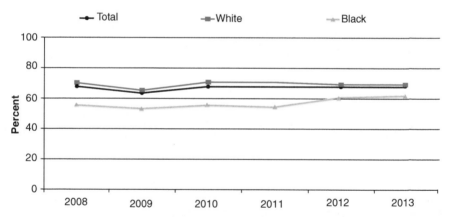

Source: Substance Abuse and Mental Health Services Administration. National Survey on Drug Use and Health. 2008–2013
Denominator: Adults age 18 and over with a major depressive episode in the past year
Note: Major depressive episode is defined as a period of at least 2 weeks when a person experienced a depressed mood or loss of interest or pleasure in daily activities and had a majority of the symptoms of depression described in the forth edition of the *Diagnostic and Statistical Manual of Mental Disorders.* Treatment for depression is defined as seeing or talking to a medical doctor or other professional or using prescription medication in the past year for depression

Fig. 12.1 Adults with a major depressive episode in the past year who received treatment for depression in the past year, by race, 2008–2013. Chartbook on Health Care for Blacks: National Healthcare Quality and Disparities Report. https://www.ahrq.gov/research/findings/nhqrdr/chartbooks/blackhealth/acknow.html

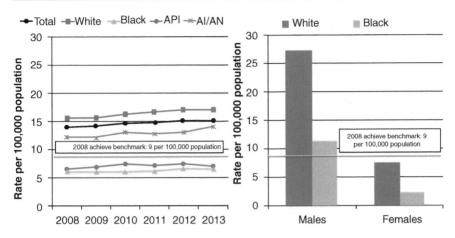

Key: API = Asian or Pacific Islander: AI/AN = American Indian or Alaska Native
Source: Centers for Disease Control and Prevention. National Center for Health Statistics.
National Vital Statistics System-Mortality. 2008-2013
Note: For this measure, lower rates are better. Estimates are age adjusted to the 2000
U.S standard population

Fig. 12.2 Suicide deaths per 100,000 population, by race, 2008–2013, and stratified by sex for Blacks and Whites, 2013. Chartbook on Health Care for Blacks: National Healthcare Quality and Disparities Report. https://www.ahrq.gov/research/findings/nhqrdr/chartbooks/blackhealth/acknow.html

> behaviors (e.g., smoking, alcohol use and abuse, drug use, and overeating, especially of comfort foods) that help to alleviate the resulting symptoms of stress. However, these same behaviors silently contribute to physical health morbidities and early mortality. [16]

Their hypothesis suggests that by activating the hypothalamic axis through alcohol, smoking, pleasure foods, illegal stimulants, and other illicit drugs, African Americans directly alleviate the symptoms of the stressor but also do irreparable damage to their long-term physical health:

> (African) American women show heightened rates of obesity over the life course. Overeating is an effective, early, well-learned response to chronic environmental stressors that only strengthens over the life course. In contrast, for a variety of social and cultural reasons, (African) American men's coping choices and trajectories are different from that of (African American) women's. Early in life, (African American) men tend to lead active, athletic lives, but in middle age the viability and effectiveness of this dopamine-producing coping strategy is reduced because of physical deterioration. It is at middle age that (African American) men begin to show increased rates of smoking, alcohol consumption, and illicit drug use. [13]

Other studies relating to mental health in African Americans confirm the increased incidence of having concurrent chronic physical health conditions (cardiovascular disease or diabetes) in addition to existing mood or anxiety disorders.

African Americans have increased comorbidities, so it is also understandable that if there is mental illness, comorbidities would coexist as well.

The legitimacy of Jackson's theory would hold better if there were confirmed higher substance use and abuse in African Americans, but there is not. Leah Wilty at Northwestern University looked at drug and alcohol use disorders in youths over a 12-year period:

> We found striking racial/ethnic differences. Contrary to popular stereotypes of African Americans, the prevalence of drug-use disorders such as cocaine and hallucinogen or PCP was lowest among African Americans, followed by Hispanics, then non-Hispanic Whites. For example, non-Hispanic Whites had more than 30 times the odds of having cocaine-use disorder than African Americans. [14]

The disparities in illicit drug use shrink as African Americans age, but related suicides and personal impact from drugs remain higher in European Americans.

Despite the lower prevalence of depression in African Americans, there are still significant areas of concern. When African Americans have depression, the symptoms are more severe and persistent and usually go untreated [18]. Williams and colleagues at the Institute for Social Research at the University of Michigan looked at depression in African Americans, Caribbean-born African Americans, and European Americans and summarized their findings:

> We found that both black populations with MDD (major depressive disorder) were over-represented among persons with very severe impairment, with African Americans having higher levels than Caribbean blacks on some indicators of impairment. Blacks with severe impairment, irrespective of ethnicity, reported substantially more days out of role than the national average for persons with MDD. These data suggest that when blacks develop MDD, it is likely debilitating in impact and persistent in its course. It is important to find out why blacks who develop this illness have a poorer prognosis than their white counterparts. These findings also emphasize the need for the treatment of blacks with MDD. In the United States, 57% of adults with MDD receive treatment, but we found that most blacks with MDD, irrespective of ethnicity, do not receive treatment. Only 48% of African Americans and 22% of Caribbean blacks with severe symptoms received treatment. [23]

As providers, remember to keep depression in mind as a driver for a number of other complaints that African American patients may report. Suggest that insomnia, fatigue, overeating, and an array of other complaints may be a manifestation of depression. Trust, time, and education will help them agree to treatment.

As alluded to earlier, African Americans are much more likely to be diagnosed with a schizophrenia-spectrum diagnosis (psychoses) than an affective diagnosis (depression, bipolar, anxiety) when compared to European Americans

[24–26]. Schwartz and colleagues explored two possibilities as the cause: epigenetic differences by race or a systematic and consistent error or bias in the diagnostic process:

> The present study found that African Americans were diagnosed with a schizophrenia-spectrum diagnosis at a higher rate than (European American) individuals, which was also evident in the rate of (European American) individuals diagnosed with an affective disorder compared with African Americans. More important, no differences in symptoms were found. [25]

The authors proposed that making a diagnosis is based on a constellation of symptoms, and while the symptoms might be the same between an African American and a European American patient, the final diagnosis involves a "higher level" of reasoning. Diagnoses, they suggest, "reflect a global, overall impression, that includes multiple streams of information including behavioral observation but also historical information and collateral report" [25]. These added "considerations" lead to skewed diagnostic outcomes and lasting stigmatization. These overdiagnosed patients carry the added burden of the diagnosis and the side-effect profile of whatever antipsychotic medication was started.

Your approach to a new patient with a history of schizophrenia may be different from an approach to the same patient with a history of depression; if the patient is African American, consider overdiagnosis as a possibility.

12.3   Increased Exposure to Death

One of the more serious life stresses is the death of a family member. Debra Umberson and colleagues at the University of Texas at Austin outlined the significantly increased exposure to the death of a parent, spouse, or child and its impact on the African American psyche and health [27]:

> This study provides a population-based documentation of earlier and repeated bereavement experiences for (African) Americans, who are more likely to experience the deaths of mothers, fathers, siblings, spouses, and children and to experience multiple family member deaths. Moreover, racial differences in exposure to death of mothers, fathers, and siblings appear early in childhood. By early to mid-adulthood, racial differences in exposure to the death of children and spouses are also significant. Understanding exposure to family deaths from childhood through mid to later life is important because bereavement experiences almost certainly add to cumulative disadvantage in multiple life outcomes. Past research has generally focused on the effects of only one loss on subsequent life outcomes, clearly demonstrating adverse effects of bereavement on socioeconomic status, mental health, health behaviors, physical health, and mortality risk. [27]

The death of only one critical family member has been shown to negatively impact the life course of an individual. African Americans, for medical reasons we have already reviewed, deal with multiple deaths of critical family and friends throughout their lives, burying parents, siblings, spouses, and offspring. The psychiatric burden should be, and is, great, but for "whatever reason" acceptance prevails.

12.4   Alcohol

Alcohol consumption among the races, based on the "National Survey on Drug Use and Health" data, range from European Americans at almost 57% using alcohol to a low among Asian Americans at 40%. African American alcohol consumption rests at 44% of the racial population [28].

In African Americans, the number of underage drinkers is low and there is also low reported heavy on-going alcohol use [29]. A higher number report episodic binge drinking, and this behavior adds to higher social consequences in African Americans. Because of the lower drinking in adolescence, African Americans have fewer earlier age DUIs but catch up later in life and ultimately show higher social consequences of drinking [30]. Particularly, there is a higher male-to-female and female-to-male intimate partner violence reported [31].

One important medical consequence of alcohol in African Americans is liver cirrhosis. African Americans have a greater risk for developing alcohol-related liver disease than European Americans [32]. Additionally, rates of alcohol-related esophageal cancer and pancreatic disease are also higher for African American men than European American men [33].

12.5   Sleep Differences

There are also racial disparities in sleep with African Americans having "shorter sleep duration, greater onset latency, and higher awakening after sleep onset" [34]. There was also a decreased ability to phase shift African Americans sleep cycles when exposed to jet-lag and shift work situations, and the total duration of the cycle was smaller, a study by Eastman and colleagues at Rush University Medical Center found [35].

These researchers surmised that the differences in sleep architecture grew from thousands of years of genetic modifications resulting from, for Africans, exposure to year-around consistent 12-hour light-dark cycles, versus Europeans coming for northern regions with significant variability in the day length, dawn, and dusk times. The shifting circadian periods in non-equatorial regions instilled a genetically modified increased tolerance for variable light-dark productivity hours:

The magnitude and direction of the phase shift was related to the free-running circadian period, and European-Americans had a longer circadian period than African-Americans. Circadian period was related to the percent Sub-Saharan African and European ancestry from DNA samples. We speculate that a short circadian period was advantageous during our evolution in Africa and lengthened with northern migrations out of Africa. The differences in circadian rhythms remaining today are relevant for understanding and treating the modern circadian-rhythm-based disorders which are due to a misalignment between the internal circadian rhythms and the times for sleep, work, school and meals. [35]

In another study, Eastman exposed African Americans and European Americans to a 9-hour delayed light-dark sleep-wake and meal schedule, similar to traveling from Chicago to Japan [36]. Essentially what would take 10 days for full adjustment in European Americans would take 15 days for African Americans to adjust. The need to adjust to time zone changes is only periodic in most people, and there are methods to make this adjustment smoother, but shift work seen in factory workers, police and fire positions, healthcare staff, and other positions place an additional health burden on these workers. Shift working was found to add an additional 40% risk of cardiovascular disease as compared to non-shift work [37]. There is increased obesity as a result of decreased glucose tolerance from meals consumed in the night, as well as elevated triglycerides and lowered HDL levels … all contributing to increased morbidity and mortality [37].

Shift work is more prevalent in the African American community and is associated with worse health outcomes including increased smoking, elevated blood pressures, obesity, increased alcohol use, decreased physical activity, depression, and work stress [38]. Getting a thorough work history and looking for shift work and then counseling and screening for these increased disease propensities can provide a significant benefit for your patient. By incorporating a planned exercise schedule and diet, reaffirming the dangers of smoking (particularly in shift workers), and providing better insight into the social impact of these schedules, many of the detriments of shift work can be tempered. And the few individuals that continually fail to adjust to shift work may find solace in the possible existence of a genetic inability to ever adjust.

12.6 Vitamin and Supplements

Vitamin D is acquired through diet and skin exposure to ultraviolet B light. The skin's production of vitamin D is determined by length of exposure, latitude, season, and degree of skin pigmentation. African Americans produce less vitamin D3 than do European Americans in response to matched levels of sun exposure and have dramatically lower 25-hydroxyvitamin D [25(OH)D] concentrations with some studies indicating up to 96% of the African American population as deficient [39]. Yet both races tend to have similar capacities to absorb vitamin D and to produce vitamin D when exposed to light [40].

Overall when measured, African Americans tend to have lower vitamin D3 levels and are very frequently labeled vitamin D deficient but also have confirmed stronger bones and fewer fractures. Powe and colleagues at the Brigham and Woman's Hospital in Cambridge Massachusetts looked specifically at this paradox as it related to vitamin D3- and vitamin D-binding proteins [40].

> Lower levels of vitamin D–binding protein in blacks appear to result in levels of bioavailable 25-hydroxyvitamin D that are equivalent to those in whites. These data … suggest that low total 25-hydroxyvitamin D levels do not uniformly indicate vitamin D deficiency and call into question routine supplementation in persons with low levels of both total 25-hydroxyvitamin D and vitamin D– binding protein who lack other traditional manifestations of this condition. [40]

Vitamin D

Twenty to thirty minutes of midday sun exposure two to three times a week on the face and forearms can generate up to 2000 IU of vitamin D in lighter skin-pigmented persons. Higher pigmented skin may require 2–10 times more sun exposure compared to lighter completion individuals and may not be a reasonable recommendation. For this population, vitamin D supplementation is the answer.

The result of these studies suggests that having both a low vitamin D3 level and a low vitamin D-binding protein in African Americans actually causes a "reset" of true deficiency. With both being low, it is vitamin D3's bioavailability that drives calcium levels, parathyroid hormone levels, and true bone risk.

Dr. Powe concluded:

> Vitamin D deficiency is certainly present in persons with very low levels of total 25-hydroxyvitamin D accompanied by hyperparathyroidism, hypocalcemia, or low BMD (bone mass density). However, community-dwelling (African Americans) with total 25-hydroxyvitamin D levels below the threshold used to define vitamin D deficiency typically lack these accompanying characteristic alterations. The high prevalence among (African Americans) of a polymorphism in the vitamin D–binding protein gene that is associated with low levels of vitamin D–binding protein results in levels of bioavailable 25-hydroxyvitamin D that are similar to those in (European Americans), despite lower

levels of total 25-hydroxyvitamin D. Alterations in vitamin D–binding protein levels may therefore be responsible for observed racial differences in total 25-hydroxyvitamin D levels and manifestations of vitamin D deficiency. [40]

But wait … do not stop suggesting vitamin D supplementation yet! Ken Batai and colleagues at the University of Arizona, through studying over 2000 patients, found a direct benefit to vitamin D supplementation to preventing prostate cancer in African American men and a pro-carcinogenic effect of calcium supplementation on the prostate [41]. These findings were strongest in African Americans:

Calcium and vitamin D are important nutrients, and they may have preventive effects against many health conditions. Although toxicity from high vitamin D supplementation may be low, high calcium intake is associated with increased prostate cancer risk as well as risk of cardiovascular disease and kidney stones. High calcium consumption might be harmful and for prostate cancer prevention, high dose calcium supplementation and fortification should be avoided, especially among (African American) men. [41]

If your African American patient is concerned about prostate cancer, vitamin D supplementation may be of help … and if your patient is a health nut on multiple supplements, or has heartburn and takes a lot of antacids, check to insure the calcium supplementation is not overly aggressive. High calcium intake in African American men may actually increase the risk for prostate cancer.

Vitamin D measurement and appropriate supplementation in African American patients with renal insufficiency have been suggested by the National Kidney Foundation due to its beneficial effects [42]. With the increased kidney disease in African Americans and the concomitant lower vitamin D levels across the African American population, the benefits of vitamin D replacement in these patients are high. Lunyera and colleagues at Duke University looked vitamin D and chronic kidney disease in the Jackson Heart Study [43].

Our data also support a role of low 25(OH)D as an independent risk for faster decline in kidney function in (African) Americans with diabetes. This finding corroborates, in an exclusively (African American) cohort, a growing body of evidence that suggests low 25(OH)D confers greater risk factor for adverse CKD outcomes among individuals with diabetic kidney disease. [43]

Another study linked vitamin D level to the patient's risk for ovarian cancer:

The role of Vitamin D in human cancers, including ovarian cancer, has been widely investigated, where it was proposed to play a protective and antitumorigenic role by regulating cellular proliferation and metabolism. In this review, we have shown that vitamin D status may be an independent predictor of prognosis in ovarian cancer patients. Vitamin D combination therapy improves antitumor effects allowing for potential clinical application. Supplement of vitamin D and calcium combination may be an efficient method for cancer prevention. [44]

Yao and Ambrosone looked at the association between vitamin D deficiency and aggressive breast cancer in African American women and found [45]:

The relationship of vitamin D with breast cancer risk may be subtype-specific, with emerging evidence of stronger effects of vitamin D for more aggressive breast cancer, particularly in women of African ancestry. [45]

A link between vitamin D and colon cancer exists as well [46]:

our work provides evidence of differences in transcriptional responses to a fixed dose of (vitamin D) $1\alpha,25(OH)_2D_3$ between African Americans and European Americans … These inter-ethnic response differences are irrespective of serum 25(OH)D levels suggesting that even if equivalent serum levels are achieved between populations, there could still be differences in response at the tissue level. We provide evidence supporting a genetic mechanism underlying inter-ethnic differences in vitamin D … [46]

Sannette Hall and Devendra Agrawal at Creighton University examined the studies regarding vitamin D and asthma, and while they did not find firm evidence that vitamin D replacement helps, they had clear recommendations [47]:

Several epidemiological and *in vivo* studies have found a link between low serum levels of vitamin D and increased inflammation, decline in lung function, increased exacerbations and overall poor outcome in patients with asthma. Although vitamin D supplementation has appeared to be a viable option for adjunct therapy, results from clinical trials have primarily shown that supplementation has very little, if any, effect on improvement of symptoms or onset of asthma in patients. It is important to note that these clinical trials are not without limitations. Limited sample sizes as well as variations in dosage and the duration of trials are all factors which may have contributed to some of the observed results. Clearly, there is still a great deal of work to be done in the field. Studies are first needed to clearly define the most optimal technique for measuring serum vitamin D levels and arrive at some consensus for what is described as vitamin D deficiency and insufficiency. Additionally, future research needs to identify the optimal dose of vitamin D for distinct groups based on gender, ethnicity, age, cultural practices and asthmatic phenotype since all these factors affect absorption and available levels of vitamin D. [47]

The increased occurrence of asthma in African Americans coupled with worse outcomes and incomplete recommendations as it relates to African Americans makes supplementation with vitamin D a reasonable default until more definitive information is available.

Aside from vitamin D, vitamin and mineral deficiencies in African Americans have largely been linked to dietary, cultural, and socioeconomic differences [48]. Some of these deficiencies have been linked to the increased occurrence of hypertension, cardiovascular disease, diabetes, breast cancer, colon cancer, ovarian cancer, kidney disease, and more [48, 49]. Curiously, many of these studies found associations in one racial group but not another. Increased calcium was associated with prostate cancer in African Americans but not European Americans [41]. Vitamin D replacement was associated with lower breast cancer rates in African American woman but not European American women [45].

Vitamin D Deficiency: Possible Link
- Prostate cancer
- Renal insufficiency
- Ovarian cancer
- Breast cancer
- Colon cancer
- Asthma susceptibility

Researchers initially believed selenium and vitamin E were the key to decreased prostate cancer, but a large well-designed study refuted that hypothesis [50, 51]. In fact, outcomes suggested that vitamin E supplementation actually caused more prostate cancer.

Because of superior renal conservation of calcium, African Americans require 300 mg less calcium per day than European Americans [52, 53]. Researchers hypothesize that the lower 25-hydroxyvitamin D levels drive up the parathyroid hormone levels leading to reduced loss of calcium through the kidneys. The reduced loss leads to reduced need in African Americans [53].

Edward Suarez and Nicole Schramm-Sapyta at Duke University looked for racial differences related to vitamins A, C, and E and β-carotene to metabolic and inflammatory biomarkers and determined a link between β-carotene and insulin resistance [54]:

Among African Americans, lower β-carotene levels were associated with higher estimates of insulin resistance and fasting insulin; whereas, these same associations were not significant for whites. Race also significantly moderated the relation of vitamin C to leukocyte count, with lower vitamin C being associated with higher leukocyte count only in African Americans but not (European Americans). For all subjects, lower β-carotene was associated with higher high sensitivity C-reactive protein. In African Americans, but not (European

Americans), lower levels of β-carotene and vitamin C were significantly associated with
early risk markers implicated in cardiometabolic conditions and cancer. [54]

Lower β-carotene levels have also been associated with an increased risk for colon
cancer and non-Hodgkin lymphoma [55, 56]. C-reactive protein has long been associated with worse cardiovascular outcomes and cardiometabolic conditions [57, 58].
Insufficient B vitamin levels (and folate) have also been associated with elevated
stroke risk, which is also overrepresented in the African American population [59].

The common theme throughout this research highlights the importance of tailoring essential vitamin and mineral supplementation to the patient's needs.

Vitamin Deficiencies: Possible Link

Vitamin B6	Stroke
Vitamin B2 (Riboflavin)	Stroke
Folate	Anemia
	Dementia
Zinc	Prostate cancer
β-Carotene	Insulin resistance
	Colon cancer
	Non-Hodgkin lymphoma

12.7   Bone Health

It has been well established that African Americans have fewer bone fractures across
their lifetime [60–63]. Fewer fractures in African Americans have been linked to
higher bone mass density and more favorable bone microarchitecture including
greater cortical thickness and higher trabecular density. These differences increase
bone strength by conferring added resistance to bending and twisting forces that
could lead to fractures [64]. African Americans also have "certain bone histomor-
phometric and geometric features and fall patterns that also could protect them from
fractures" [65].

The prevalence of osteoporosis and osteopenia is consistently lower in African
Americans compared to European Americans [66]. Lynn Marshall and the
Osteoporotic Fractures in Men Research Group looked at the volumetric bone
mass density of over 3000 African Americans, Asian Americans, Hispanic/Latino
Americans, and European Americans that were over 65 years of age looking for
structural differences in femoral neck bone strength [64]. They found that African
Americans had greater bone density, larger cortical volume, and greater cortical
thickness. The African American men in the study of similar height also had a
higher body mass index.

The overall 50% decreased risk for fracture in African Americans is significant, but there are millions of fractures in the USA every year, and a significant number still occur in this population. The number of African Americans with preventable fractures still represents a significant population that needs to be screened, advised, and possibly treated. As the number of older African Americans grows, so will the number at risk for fracture [60]. A study by Hamrick and colleagues at the Brody School of Medicine found a significantly smaller proportion of African American women compared to European American woman treated for osteoporosis once it was diagnosed. They suggest that the decreased treatment in the face of a confirmed diagnosis stems "from an illogical application of evidence that African Americans are at lower risk of osteoporosis" [67]. The overall lower risk for osteoporosis is wrongly attributed to *every* African American, even those with a confirmed diagnosis of osteoporosis. Every patient with osteoporosis should be treated appropriately.

12.8 Vaccinations

African Americans are less likely to accept vaccinations of any kind with data showing over 50% of adults refusing [68]. Vicki Freimuth and colleagues looked at the determinants of trust in the flu vaccine for African Americans and confirmed that basic trust is still at the root of this disparity [69]:

> In the United States today, there is frequently highly polarized public discourse on vaccines in general, and particularly for children, with anti-vaccine groups setting a negative tone about vaccines. Although much of that discourse focuses on children, it can feed a broader skepticism about vaccines, including the flu vaccine. Racial dynamics are also a critical factor in shaping vaccine trust, with African Americans expressing lower trust in the flu vaccine and the vaccine process than (European American) adults. Given that the longstanding racial disparity in influenza immunization places African American adults at risk for influenza-related morbidity and mortality, strengthening trust in the flu vaccine and the vaccine process is critically important in increasing vaccine uptake. Our results suggest that strategic and targeted messages from health care providers and public health agencies can facilitate improved trust. [69]

Frequently those who refuse vaccinations do so because of false perceptions regarding side effects including the belief that the shot itself will make them sick. Some attribute any illness after the vaccination to a poor outcome from the vaccination, and still others attribute more conspiracy-related theories.

Important differences in the clinical care of patients are discovered every day. As researchers tease out the significance of the more important differences, clinicians will need to be nimble in their review and discerning in their implementation. Disparities exist because there are differences. Quality care prevails when we recognize differences and adjust accordingly.

Other Important Differences

- African Americans have greater pain sensitivity and lower pain tolerance but receive a lesser quality of pain care.
- African Americans are more likely to have their pain discounted or under-estimated and less likely to be screened for pain.
- African Americans show a consistent decreased occurrence of opioid-related abuse.
- African Americans have fewer mental illnesses with significantly less anxiety, depression, and suicide than other populations.
- When African Americans have depression, the symptoms are more severe and persistent and are more resistant to treatment.
- African Americans are much more likely to be diagnosed with a schizophrenia-spectrum diagnosis (psychoses) than an affective diagnosis (depression, bipolar, anxiety) when compared to European Americans.
- The prevalence of drug use disorders was lowest among African Americans with European Americans having 30 times the odds of having a cocaine-related disorder.
- African Americans have a greater risk for developing *alcohol-related* liver disease, esophageal cancer, and pancreatic disease than European Americans.
- African Americans have shorter sleep duration, greater onset latency, and higher awakening after sleep onset.
- African Americans have a decreased tolerance for jet lag and shift work.
- Even though African Americans have lower vitamin D concentrations than European Americans, the levels of bioavailable vitamin D are similar to those of European Americans.
- Vitamin D deficiency has been linked to cancers of the prostate, ovary, breast, and colon.
- Vitamin D deficiency has also been linked to renal insufficiency and increased asthma susceptibility.
- African Americans have stronger bones and fewer fractures than European Americans despite the lower levels of vitamin D.
- Vitamin D supplementation may be of benefit to preventing prostate cancer in African American males.
- In African American men, high calcium intake is associated with increased prostate cancer risk as well as risk for cardiovascular disease and kidney stones.

- Vitamin D measurement and supplementation in African American patients with renal disease are suggested by the National Kidney Foundation.
- African Americans have fewer bone fractures and less osteoporosis and osteopenia.
- Fewer fractures in African Americans have been linked to higher bone mass density and more favorable bone microarchitecture including greater cortical thickness and higher trabecular density.
- African Americans are less likely to accept vaccinations of any kind.

References

1. Edwards R, Doleys D, Fillingim R, Lowery D. Ethnic differences in pain tolerance: clinical implications in a chronic pain population. Psychosom Med. 2001;63(2):316–23. https://doi.org/10.1097/00006842-200103000-00018.
2. Campbell C, Edwards R, Fillingim R. Ethnic differences in responses to multiple experimental pain stimuli. Pain. 2005;113(1):20–6. https://doi.org/10.1016/j.pain.2004.08.013.
3. Bhimani R, Cross L, Taylor B, et al. Taking ACTION to reduce pain: ACTION study rationale, design and protocol of a randomized trial of a proactive telephone-based coaching intervention for chronic musculoskeletal pain among African Americans. BMC Musculoskelet Disord. 2017;18(1):15. https://doi.org/10.1186/s12891-016-1363-6.
4. Institute of Medicine (US) Committee on Advancing Pain Research, Care, and Education. Relieving pain in America: A blueprint for transforming prevention, care, education, and research. Washington, DC: National Academies Press; 2011. Retrieved November 22, 2018, from https://www.ncbi.nlm.nih.gov/books/NBK92516/#ch2.s5.
5. Lord B, Khalsa S. Influence of patient race on administration of analgesia by student paramedics. BMC Emerg Med. 2019;19(1):32.
6. Ringwall C, Gugelmann H, Garrettson M, et al. Differential prescribing of opioid analgesics according to physician specialty for Medicaid patients with chronic noncancer pain diagnoses. Pain Res Manag. 2014;19(4):179–85.
7. Anderson K, Green C, Payne R. Racial and ethnic disparities in pain: causes and consequences of unequal care. J Pain. 2009;10(12):1187–204. https://doi.org/10.1016/j.jpain.2009.10.002.
8. Goyal M, Kuppermann N, Cleary S, Teach S, Chamberlain J. Racial disparities in pain management of children with appendicitis in emergency departments. JAMA Pediatr. 2015;169(11):996. https://doi.org/10.1001/jamapediatrics.2015.1915.
9. Meghani S, Byun E, Gallagher R. Time to take stock: a meta-analysis and systematic review of analgesic treatment disparities for pain in the United States. Pain Med. 2012;13(2):150–74. https://doi.org/10.1111/j.1526-4637.2011.01310.x.
10. Shavers V, Bakos A, Sheppard V. Race, ethnicity, and pain among the U.S. adult population. J Health Care Poor Underserved. 2010;21(1):177–220. https://doi.org/10.1353/hpu.0.0255.

11. Ringwalt C, Roberts A, Gugelmann H, Skinner A. Racial disparities across provider specialties in opioid prescriptions dispensed to Medicaid beneficiaries with chronic noncancer pain. Pain Med. 2015;16(4):633–40. https://doi.org/10.1111/pme.12555.

12. Feng J, Iser J, Yang W. Medical encounters for opioid-related intoxications in Southern Nevada: sociodemographic and clinical correlates. BMC Health Serv Res. 2016;16(1):438. https://doi.org/10.1186/s12913-016-1692-z.

13. Burgess D, Crowley-Matoka M, Phelan S, et al. Patient race and physician's decisions to prescribe opioids for chronic low back pain. Soc Sci Med. 2008;67(11):1852–60. https://doi.org/10.1016/j.socscimed.2008.09.009.

14. Johnson-Lawrence V, Griffith D, Watkins D. The effects of race, ethnicity, and mood/anxiety disorders on the chronic physical health conditions of men from a national sample. Am J Mens Health. 2013;7(4_suppl):58S–67S. https://doi.org/10.1177/1557988313484960.

15. Hankerson SH, Suite D, Bailey RK. Treatment disparities among African American men with depression: implications for clinical practice. J Health Care Poor Underserved. 2015;26(1):21–34.

16. Jackson J, Knight K, Rafferty J. Race and unhealthy behaviors: chronic stress, the HPA Axis, and physical and mental health disparities over the life course. Am J Public Health. 2010;100(5):933–9. https://doi.org/10.2105/ajph.2008.143446.

17. Breslau J, Kendler KS, Su M, et al. Lifetime risk and persistence of psychiatric disorders across ethnic groups in the United States. Psychol Med. 2005;35(3):317–27.

18. Breslau J, Aguilar-Gaxiola S, Kendler KS, et al. Specifying race-ethnic differences in risk for psychiatric disorder in a USA national sample. Psychol Med. 2006;36(1):57–68.

19. Barnes DM, Bates LM. Do racial patterns in psychological distress shed light on the Black-White depression paradox? A systematic review. Soc Psychiatry Psychiatr Epidemiol. 2017;52(8):913–28.

20. Whaley AL. Effects of gender- matching and racial self- labeling on paranoia in African American men with severe mental illness. J Natl Med Assoc. 2006;98(4):551–8.

21. Suite DH, La Bril R, Primm A, Harrison-Ross P. Beyond misdiagnosis, misunderstanding and mistrust: relevance of the historical perspective in the medical and mental health treatment of people of color. J Natl Med Assoc. 2007;99(8):879–85.

22. Chartbook on health care for blacks. Rockville: Agency for Healthcare Research and Quality. https://www.ahrq.gov/research/findings/nhqrdr/chartbooks/blackhealth/acknow.html.

23. Williams DR, Gonzalez HM, Neighbors H, et al. Prevalence and distribution of major depressive disorder in African Americans, Caribbean blacks, and non-Hispanic whites: results from the National Survey of American Life. Arch Gen Psychiatry. 2007;64(3):305–15.

24. Minsky S, Vega W, Miskimen T, et al. Diagnostic patterns in Latino, African American, and European American psychiatric patients. Arch Gen Psychiatry. 2003;60(6):637–44.

25. Schwartz EK, Docherty NM, Najolia GM, Cohen AS. Exploring the racial diagnostic bias of schizophrenia using behavioral and clinical-based measures. J Abnorm Psychol. 2019;128(3):263–71.

26. Olbert CM, Nagendra A, Buck B. Meta-analysis of Black vs. White racial disparity in schizophrenia diagnosis in the United States: do structured assessments attenuate racial disparities? J Abnormal Psychol. 2018;127(1):104–15.

27. Umberson D, Olson J, Crosnoe R, Liu H, Pudrovska T, Donnelly R. Death of family members as an overlooked source of racial disadvantage in the United States. Proc Natl Acad Sci. 2017;114(5):915–20.

28. Substance Abuse and Mental Health Services Administration. Key substance use and mental health indicators in the United States: Results from the 2016 National Survey on Drug Use and Health (HHS Publication No. SMA 17-5044, NSDUH Series H-52). Rockville: Center for Behavioral Health Statistics and Quality, Substance Abuse and Mental Health Services Administration; 2017. Retrieved from https://www.samhsa.gov/data/.

29. Chartier K, Hesselbrock M, Hesselbrock V. Ethnicity and adolescent pathways to alcohol use. J Stud Alcohol Drugs. 2009;70(3):337–45. https://doi.org/10.15288/jsad.2009.70.337.

30. Welty L, Harrison A, Abram K, et al. Health disparities in drug- and alcohol-use disorders: a 12-year longitudinal study of youths after detention. Am J Public Health. 2016;106(5):872–80. https://doi.org/10.2105/ajph.2015.303032.

31. Caetano R, Cunradi C, Schafer J, Clark C. Intimate partner violence and drinking patterns among white, black, and hispanic couples in the U.S. J Subst Abus. 2000;11(2):123–38. https://doi.org/10.1016/s0899-3289(00)00015-8.

32. Flores Y, Yee H, Leng M, et al. Risk factors for chronic liver disease in blacks, Mexican Americans, and Whites in the United States: results from NHANES IV, 1999–2004. Am J Gastroenterol. 2008;103(9):2231–8. https://doi.org/10.1111/j.1572-0241.2008.02022.x.

33. Polednak A. Secular trend in U.S. Black-White disparities in selected alcohol-related cancer incidence rates. Alcohol Alcohol. 2007;42(2):125–30. https://doi.org/10.1093/alcalc/agl121.

34. Fuller-Rowell T, Curtis D, El-Sheikh M, Chae D, Boylan J, Ryff C. Racial disparities in sleep: the role of neighborhood disadvantage. Sleep Med. 2016;27–28:1–8. https://doi.org/10.1016/j.sleep.2016.10.008.

35. Eastman C, Suh C, Tomaka V, Crowley S. Circadian rhythm phase shifts and endogenous free-running circadian period differ between African-Americans and European-Americans. Sci Rep. 2015;5(1):8381. https://doi.org/10.1038/srep08381.

36. Eastman C, Tomaka V, Crowley S. Circadian rhythms of European and African-Americans after a large delay of sleep as in jet lag and night work. Sci Rep. 2016;6(1):36716. https://doi.org/10.1038/srep36716.

37. Knutsson A. Health disorders of shift workers. Occup Med. 2003;53(2):103–8. https://doi.org/10.1093/occmed/kqg048.

38. Books C, Coody LC, Kauffman R, Abraham S. Night shift work and its health effects on nurses. Health Care Manag. 2017;36(4):347–53.

39. Holick M, Binkley N, Bischoff-Ferrari H, et al. Evaluation, treatment, and prevention of vitamin D deficiency: an endocrine society clinical practice guideline. J Clin Endocrinol Metab. 2011;96(7):1911–30. https://doi.org/10.1210/jc.2011-0385.

40. Powe C, Evans M, Wenger J, et al. Vitamin D–binding protein and vitamin D status of black Americans and white Americans. N Engl J Med. 2013;369(21):1991–2000. https://doi.org/10.1056/nejmoa1306357.

41. Batai K, Murphy A, Ruden M, et al. Race and BMI modify associations of calcium and vitamin D intake with prostate cancer. BMC Cancer. 2017;17(1):64. https://doi.org/10.1186/s12885-017-3060-8.

42. Vitamin D: The Kidney Vitamin? National Kidney Foundation. 2019. https://www.kidney.org/news/kidneyCare/spring10/VitaminD. Accessed 25 May 2019.

43. Lunyera J, Davenport CA, Pendergast J, et al. Modifiers of plasma 25-hydroxyvitamin D and chronic kidney disease outcomes in black Americans: the Jackson heart study. J Clin Endocrinol Metab. 2019;104(6):2267–76.

44. Guo H, Guo J, Xie W, et al. The role of vitamin D in ovarian cancer: epidemiology, molecular mechanism and prevention. J Ovarian Res. 2018;11:71.
45. Yao S, Ambrosone CB. Associations between vitamin D deficiency and risk of aggressive breast cancer in African American women. J Steroid Biochem Mol Biol. 2013;136:337–41.
46. Alleyne D, Witonsky D, Mapes B, et al. Colonic transcriptional response to 1α,25(OH)2 vitamin D3 in African- and European-Americans. J Steroid Biochem Mol Biol. 2017;168:49–59.
47. Hall SC, Agrawal DK. Vitamin D and bronchial asthma: an overview of the last five years. Clin Ther. 2017;39(5):917–29.
48. Blumberg JB, Frei B, Fulgoni VL, et al. Contribution of dietary supplements to nutritional adequacy in race/ethnic population subgroups in the United States. Nutrients. 2017;9(12):1295.
49. CDC, National Center for Health Statistics. Second national report on biochemical indicators of diet and nutrition in the U.S. population. 2012. https://www.cdc.gov/nutritionreport/pdf/Nutrition_Book_complete508_final.pdf. Accessed 26 May 2019.
50. Lippman SM, Klein EA, Goodman PJ, et al. Effect of selenium and vitamin E on risk of prostate cancer and other cancers: the selenium and vitamin E cancer prevention trial (SELECT). JAMA. 2009;301:39–51.
51. Nicastro HL, Dunn BK. Selenium and prostate cancer prevention: insights from the selenium and vitamin E cancer prevention trial (SELECT). Nutrients. 2013;5(4):1122–48.
52. Heaney RP. Ethnicity, bone status, and the calcium requirement. Nutr Res. 2002;22:153–78.
53. Redmond J, Jarjou LMA, Zhou B, et al. Ethnic differences in calcium, phosphate and bone metabolism. Proc Nutr Soc. 2014;73(2):340–51.
54. Suarez EC, Schramm-Sapyta NL. Race differences in the relation of vitamins A, C, E and β-carotene to metabolic and inflammatory biomarkers. Nutr Res. 2014;34(1):1–10.
55. Kabat GC, Kim MY, Sarto GE, Shikany JM, Rohan TE. Repeated measurements of serum carotenoid, retinol and tocopherol levels in relation to colorectal cancer risk in the Women's Health Initiative. Eur J Clin Nutr. 2012;66:549–54.
56. Ollberding NJ, Maskarinec G, Conroy SM, et al. Prediagnostic circulating carotenoid levels and the risk of non-Hodgkin lymphoma: the multiethnic cohort. Blood. 2012;119(24):5817–23.
57. Daniels LB. Pretenders and contenders: inflammation, C-reactive protein, and interleukin-6. J Am Heart Assoc. 2017;6(10):e007490.
58. Ridker PM, Hennekens CH, Buring JE, Rifai N. C-reactive protein and other markers of inflammation in the prediction of cardiovascular disease in women. N Engl J Med. 2000;342:836–43.
59. Sanchez_Moreno C, Jimenez_Escrig A, Martin A. Stroke: roles of B vitamins, homocysteine and antioxidants. Nutr Res Rev. 2009;22(1):49–67.
60. Bulathsinhala L, Hughes JM, McKinnon CJ, et al. Risk of stress fractures varies by race/ethnic origin in a cohort study of 1.3 million US army soldiers. J Bone Miner Res. 2017;32(7):1546–53.
61. Osteoporosis Overview. NIH osteoporosis and related bone diseases National Resource Center. 2018. https://www.bones.nih.gov/health-info/bone/osteoporosis/overview. Accessed 25 May 2019.
62. Kalkwarf HJ, Zemel BS, Gilsanz V, et al. The bone mineral density in childhood study: bone mineral content and density according to age, sex, and race. J Clin Endocrinol Metab. 2007;92:2087–99.
63. Barrett-Connor E, Siris ES, Wehren LE, et al. Osteoporosis and fracture risk in women of different ethnic groups. J Bone Miner Res. 2005;20:185–94.

64. Marshall LM, Zmuda JM, Chan BK, et al. Race and ethnic variation in proximal femur structure and BMD among older men. J Bone Miner Res. 2008;23(1):121–30.

65. Aloia JF. African Americans, 25-hydroxyvitamin D, and osteoporosis: a paradox. Am J Clin Nutr. 2008;88(2):545S–50S.

66. Pothiwala P, Evans EM, Chapman-Novakofski KM. Ethnic variation in risk for osteoporosis among women: a review of biological and behavioral factors. J Womens Health (Larchmt). 2006;15(6):709–19.

67. Hamrick I, Whetstone LM, Cummings DM. Racial disparity in treatment of osteoporosis after diagnosis. Osteoporosis Int. 2006;17(11):1653–8.

68. Flu Vaccination Coverage among Adults by Mid-November 2018, by Race/Ethnicity, National Internet Flu Survey, United States, 2018–2019 Influenza Season. CDC. https://www.cdc.gov/flu/fluvaxview/vaccination-coverage-additional-2018.htm#table2. December 2018. Accessed 25 May 2019.

69. Freimuth VS, Jamison AM, An J, et al. Determinants of trust in the flu vaccine for African Americans and whites. Soc Sci Med. 2017;193:70–9.

Dietary Differences and Ways to Impact Choices

13

13.1 Historical Perspectives

Dietary differences exist due to cultural differences that can be impacted by region, community, and socioeconomic status. African Americans, by and large, came to America by way of slave ships and originally represented the poorest of the poor. The American poor had limited dietary choices; African American slaves had even less. A significant degree of creativity went into making a meal out of the "leftovers" and discards from plantation owners and their families. Because the plantation was farmland, African Americans had access to a number of fruits and vegetables, but meats were monopolized by the landowners, and only the discarded cuts of meat were reserved for slaves.

Some of the foundations of African Americans' diet stem from these slavery days, but there are also more recent adaptations that have slowly weaved into the fabric of the African American diet. Some of the changes were economic and others more convenient and culture-related. To sum up the African American diet by only referring to slave influences is to ignore one and a half centuries of added impacts that made the African American diet what it is today. Food availability, storage, financial independence, health literacy, and a sense of history and heritage all contribute to the ever-changing components of the African American diet.

Being able to positively impact an African American patient's diet will first require a fundamental knowledge of the existing components. The basics of the African American diet mirror an American diet. The "average" meal will have meat, starch, and vegetables in varying proportions [1].

Because of the scarcity of meat as a main course in slavery days, seasoning these cooked vegetable dishes with fatty cuts of low preference meat (whether smoked or

© Springer Nature Switzerland AG 2020
G. L. Hall, *Patient-Centered Clinical Care for African Americans*,
https://doi.org/10.1007/978-3-030-26418-5_13

not) quickly became a mainstay in the African American diet. Having the lean cuts reserved exclusively for the more affluent, African Americans became accustomed to other cuts of meat. Ham hocks (tibia fibula joint in pigs), neck bones (pork neck vertebrae), ox tails (beef tail), and others became a standard way to "season" and fortify boiled vegetable dishes and beans of various types including navy beans, lima beans, and black eyed peas [2].

Now that the scarcity of meat is much less of a logistical problem, the "habit" or custom of adding meats to vegetables is now merely a standard way to cook them. String beans and collard/mustard/turnip greens almost always have a smoked (and salted) cut of meat in the pot.

Processed meat which originally represented easily stored meat (and the preserving medium frequently included salt) also found its way to African American dinner tables. For African Americans, having a gene that drives up blood pressure and kidney disease in the presence of salt is an unfortunate reality given the increased presence of salted preserved meats [3].

13.2 Dietary Components

The breakdown in terms of specific meats preferred by African Americans shows a predominance of chicken and turkey, as well as relatively more fish and pork, but less beef than European and Hispanic American diets [2] (Fig. 13.1).

Overall, African Americans eat less grains, fewer eggs, less vegetables, and much less milk, but they consume significantly more meat and fruits [2]. By increasing the amount of vegetables, particularly fresh uncooked in the form of salads, more nutritional balance can be brought to the African American diet fairly easily. The increased consumption of fish and poultry (both chicken and turkey) already represents a beneficial existing tradition [1].

Although African Americans eat relatively fewer vegetables, there are also distinct differences within this category with an increased consumption of fresh green beans, fresh cabbage, and fresh greens when compared with other vegetables [4] (Fig. 13.2).

African Americans prepare more meals "from scratch" when compared to majority of the populations. This increased home cooking leads to comparatively more purchases of cooking items including spices, seasonings, and oils and preparation items including baking powder, flour, extracts, and sugars in multiple forms [4].

The more "home cooking" done in African American kitchens leads to less consumption of pre-processed or ready-to-eat foods which is considerably beneficial. Conventionally, when people think of processed and ready-to-eat foods, they generally equate them with poor nutritional quality and lower socioeconomic status. Poti, Mendez, and colleagues looked at the nutritional value of "processed foods"

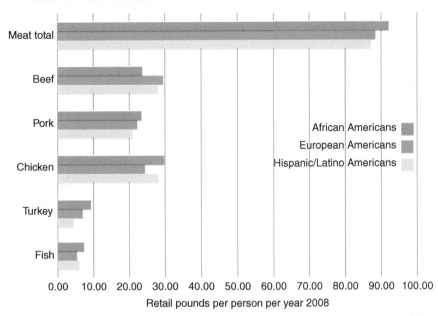

Source: USDA, Economic Research Service, calculations based on CSFII, NHANES, WWEIA, FADS and FICRCD

Fig. 13.1   Meat consumption at home by race/ethnicity. United States Department of Agriculture Economic Research Service. Commodity Consumption by Population Characteristics. (By author from raw data). https://www.ers.usda.gov/data-products/commodity-consumption-by-population-characteristics.aspx

and found they have "higher saturated fat, sugar, and sodium content" when compared to lesser processed foods [5]. Because of the higher proportion of African Americans that are poor, many assumed that they too consume more ready-to-eat foods, but studies reveal that, in fact, African Americans buy less overall ready-to-eat and/or highly processed foods when compared to European Americans [5].

One glaring exception in the purchasing of pre-processed foods was African Americans' tendency to purchase a much higher proportion of pre-processed sugary beverages when compared to European Americans and a much lower volume of milk and dairy purchases [2]. Other exceptions include a significantly higher consumption of bacon and sausages. Finally, there was also an increased purchasing of processed sweeteners including sugar, syrups, jams, and jellies in African American consumers [1].

13.3   Fried Foods

Looking at home preparation patterns, African Americans have an increased propensity to fry meats, potatoes, and other vegetables [6]. From a practical standpoint, frying foods is a fast and flavorful approach to fortifying (adding calories and substance)

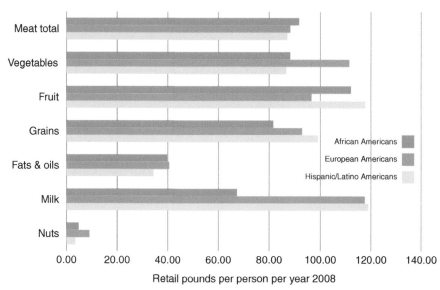

Source: USDA, Economic Research Service, calculations based on CSFII, NHANES, WWEIA, FADS and FICRCD

Fig. 13.2 Food consumption at home by race/ethnicity. United States Department of Agriculture Economic Research Service. Commodity Consumption by Population Characteristics. (By author from raw data). https://www.ers.usda.gov/data-products/commodity-consumption-by-population-characteristics.aspx

to almost any food. If you want to increase or stretch the caloric value of a food, flour or batter it, and then fry it. There is little doubt that the scarcity of food for the poor leads to practical approaches to stretching and making more palatable whatever food was present. African Americans have not just fried potatoes, but introduced fried okra, fried mushrooms, fried onions, fried green tomatoes, southern fried steak or pork chops, and a host of other dishes that started merely out of necessity. Now that there is more variety of food and it is presumably more plentiful, the "need" to fry food has diminished, but the habit and culturalization of fried foods are as strong as ever in both the African American and American-at-large communities [6].

Now that we better understand the logic behind fried foods and its place in the African American diet, decreasing the consumption due to its detrimental effects needs to be a higher priority. Sun, Lui, and colleagues at the University of Iowa looked at the impact of fried food consumption on cardiovascular mortality [6]:

> We found a significantly positive association of fried food consumption, especially fried chicken and fried fish/shellfish, with risk of all cause and cardiovascular mortality. These associations were slightly attenuated, but remained significant, after additional adjustment for a variety of factors that were related to mortality, including age, race/ethnicity, socioeconomic status, hormone use, lifestyle factors, health status, and body mass index. [6]

With obesity as a prominent public health risk and African Americans leading the way in obesity prevalence, placing fried foods as a major offender is key. Eating fried foods is dangerous from a number of perspectives. The frying process greatly increases the calorie content, increases the fat content, and significantly increases cardiovascular risk.

A lesser-known problem with frying foods is it facilitates the formation of chemical reaction by-products called advanced glycation end products (AGEs) which seem to be linked to a number of serious health issues [7]. Advanced glycation end products are the subject of ongoing research investigations into its detrimental impact on health including its promotion of cancer cell proliferation in the presence of colorectal, liver, pancreatic, and breast cancer [7]. As cooking oil is heated and used, AGEs form and become more plentiful in the oil. They are then consumed and are highly bioavailable while circulating in the body. These circulating dietary AGEs have been suspected to increase diabetes occurrence, cause premature aging, facilitate further weight gain, advance carotid stenosis and peripheral artery occlusive disease, worsen kidney disease, and promote the development and progression of heart failure [8]. All of these problems, in addition to the poor cancer outcomes, occur disproportionally in African Americans. While the research on AGEs is ongoing, and our understanding rudimentary at this point, it is fairly clear that AGEs are not at all beneficial, and while some AGEs form naturally as part of our aging process, consuming more only advances whatever pathology is present. African Americans can greatly impact the nutritional value of any meal by merely avoiding frying their foods.

Most African American patients acknowledge that fried food is bad for their health, but few know the specifics of why [9, 10]. Beyond the obvious increase in obesity (due to increased caloric content and AGE impact), increased consumption of fried foods directly leads to lower HDL cholesterol levels and higher LDL levels [11]. Increased consumption of fried foods has also been linked to the later development of type 2 diabetes and coronary heart disease [12].

Advanced Glycation End Products (AGEs)
- AGEs are generated through nonenzymatic glycation and oxidation of proteins, lipids, and nucleic acids.
- They alter tissue function and mechanical properties through cross-linking matrix proteins and through binding to their cell surface receptors.
- Enhanced formation and accumulation of AGEs have been reported to occur in conditions such as diabetes mellitus as well as in natural aging, renal failure, and chronic inflammation [8].

It should also be noted that reusing cooking oils is common in African American homes and is associated with added health risks. Heat causes oxidation and degradation of many oils with the formation of increased trans-fatty acids which have definitively been associated with increased heart disease and stroke [13]. The degradation seen with reusing oils varies based on the oil and the type of food being cooked with olive oil showing great resistance to degradation and soybean (vegetable) oils showing linear degradation with temperature and heating time [14]. Some have suggested that much of the detriment associated with increased restaurant or fast-food consumption is the prolonged and repeated use of oils and comparatively more trans-fat formation [14]. An oil with no trans-fat content can acquire significant trans-fat with heat, time, and reuse. Younger African Americans, like all Americans, find themselves eating fast food with increased frequency; advice to avoid fried fast food and giving a rationale behind the advice should improve compliance. As far as home frying is concerned, discarding oils after a "few" uses is a practical advice that is easily understood and could have a big impact.

The increased preparation of meals in the African American household also offers a big opportunity to make gradual adjustments in cooking techniques and ingredient substitutions that can have a positive impact on health over time. Making different suggestions on each patient visit can improve the adoption of healthier habits. Suggesting to not add meat to cooked vegetables, or at least substituting a lower fat content meat (e.g., switching from fatty pork meat to turkey meat), can impact health and health education. As you would discuss smoking cessation at every visit from a smoking patient, discussing small diet modifications at each visit can more reliably improve compliance and change habits.

Explaining Why Eating Fried Foods Is Bad
- Increases calorie content
- Increases obesity
- Lowers HDL cholesterol and raises LDL cholesterol
- Increases risk for type 2 diabetes
- Increases risk for heart disease
- Adds dietary AGEs
- Increases trans-fatty acids with repeated oil use

13.4   Importance of Breakfast

African Americans more frequently skip breakfast [15, 16]. The reasons range from busy schedules, the added preparation time for an "old-style breakfast" (that could include bacon, sausage, potatoes, pancakes, etc.), or the lack of an appetite. The absence of breakfast has been associated with decreased calcium, dairy, fiber, and fruit consumption [17].

Generally, the percentage of young African American children that eat breakfast starts relatively high, but that number decreases in the teen years [17]. Studies have verified that routinely eating breakfast frequently leads to more regular eating habits later in the day, improved exercise patterns, better cognition, and more healthful food choices [18, 19]. Those changes could result in less weight gain and contribute to a reduced BMI.

Making a positive impact on breakfast in African Americans first requires a starting definition. An agreement reported by the Journal of the Academy of Nutrition and Dietetics defined breakfast [18]:

> Breakfast is the first meal of the day that breaks the fast after the longest period of sleep and is consumed within 2–3 hours of waking; it is comprised of food or beverage from at least one food group, and may be consumed at any location. [18]

Having one consensus definition of breakfast allows for clinicians and researchers to move forward with recommendations from the same starting point. Before 2014, there were widely variable definitions of breakfast that lead to confusion when proposals for changes were made.

The same report (The Role of Breakfast in Health: Definition and Criteria for a Quality Breakfast) proposed criteria for a quality breakfast but also allowed for much more variability based on "age, sex, activity level, and individual tastes and preferences" [18]. By not specifically listing "what you should eat," the report allows for the realistic cultural differences in meals that already exist. The components of a quality breakfast take into account energy needs, nutrient requirements, food composition and food groups, portion sizes, and the presence of nutrient-dense foods and beverages [18].

Many older African Americans have the time (and inclination) to have a breakfast that includes bacon or sausage, eggs, and toast or pancakes. While from a cholesterol standpoint, this is not an ideal meal, eating a protein-rich breakfast has been shown to help satiety and promote sensible eating throughout the rest of the day [18].

Many Americans believe that skipping meals is a reasonable approach to weight loss and the meal most skipped is breakfast [20]. It is important to stress during weight counseling that there is controversy regarding the benefit or detriment of meal skipping. Krista Casazza and colleagues at the University of Alabama weighed the evidence behind this common belief:

> Beyond observational and single-meal studies, very little evidence directly supports or refutes the belief that breakfast eating affects weight. Shorter, single-meal, controlled studies have investigated the links between breakfast consumption and factors related to weight. Some evidence indicates that skipping breakfast results in partial compensation during subsequent meals. [20]

The significantly decreased consumption of milk and dairy products in the African American diet presents a potential increased health risk as "moderate evidence shows that the intake of milk and milk products is associated with a reduced risk of cardiovascular disease, type 2 diabetes, and lower blood pressure in adults" [21]. Constance Brown-Riggs in her article "Nutrition and Health Disparities: The Role of Dairy in Improving Minority Health Outcomes" summarized consensus recommendations for African Americans to consume three to four servings of low-fat dairy daily. An assessment of nutrient intake related to dairy consumption showed African Americans' intake of the required nutrients calcium, vitamin D, and potassium was all lower than European Americans and Hispanic/Latino Americans.

13.4.1 Lactose Intolerance

The choice for African Americans to avoid milk and related products is not entirely voluntary. Research has consistently shown that 75% or more of African Americans are lactose intolerant [22, 23]. Poor digestion of lactose occurs when insufficient amounts of lactase are available in the small intestine to hydrolyze lactose into its two constituents, galactose and glucose. New evidence is discovering that the proportion of people that are lactose intolerant could be tied to their region of genetic origin [24]. Put simply, regions where dairy herds could be raised safely and efficiently produced people that could digest lactose better. Harsher climates in African and Asia restricted the availability of dairy herds that produced milk and thus produced people with much more lactose intolerance, a study at Cornell University found [24]. Researchers found a wide range of lactose intolerances with as low as 2% of the population of Denmark descendants to as high as 100% of the people with Zambian origin. Their survey "found that lactose intolerance decreases with increasing latitude and increases with rising temperature" [24].

The process of replacing the missing nutrients resulting from low dairy consumption has become fairly easy due to lactase-fortified milks, as well as multiple milk equivalents including soy, almond, coconut, and others that can be used as part of a healthy breakfast. Oatmeal and/or whole grain cereals with milk equivalents can make a fast and nutritionally efficient meal.

13.5   Beverage Differences

As reviewed earlier, there is a substantial difference in the drinking practices of both teen and adult African Americans. Milk and water consumption is particularly low, while sugar-sweetened beverages (SSBs) are all significantly higher [2]. The consumption of fruit juice, soda, sport drinks, and all other sweetened beverages is significantly higher in African Americans [25–27].

An African American woman consumes almost double the sugar-sweetened beverage amounts than European American woman of the same age [26]. A historical review showed decreased consumption of sugar-sweetened beverages in the 1980s with a gradual increase to today's significant surplus [25]. Several studies link the trend directly to targeted and financially disproportional marketing of sugar-sweetened beverages to African Americans [25, 28, 29].

The over-consumption of sugar-sweetened beverages doesn't start in childhood, in fact European American male children and teens consume more sweetened beverages when compared to African American males of similar ages, but somewhere in their twenties, European Americans decrease their consumption and African Americans increase consumption [26] (Fig. 13.3).

Looking at African American women in particular, there is an across-the-board increased average daily consumption from sugar-sweetened beverages. The Black

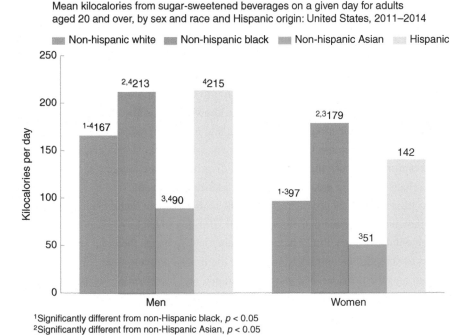

Mean kilocalories from sugar-sweetened beverages on a given day for adults aged 20 and over, by sex and race and Hispanic origin: United States, 2011–2014

■ Non-hispanic white ■ Non-hispanic black ■ Non-hispanic Asian   Hispanic

[1]Significantly different from non-Hispanic black, $p < 0.05$
[2]Significantly different from non-Hispanic Asian, $p < 0.05$
[3]Significantly different from Hispanic, $p < 0.05$
[4]Significantly different from women, $p < 0.05$
NOTE: Access data table for Figure 3 at: https://www.cdc.gov/nchs/data/databriefs/db270_table.pdf#3
SOURCE: NCHS, National Health and Nutririon Examination Survey, 2011–2014

Fig. 13.3 Daily calories from sugar-sweetened beverages by race/ethnicity and sex. https://www.cdc.gov/nchs/data/databriefs/db270.pdf

Women's Health Study found that women who transitioned from drinking "one or fewer soft drinks per week to drinking one or more soft drinks per day" saw the greatest weight gain (15 pounds) [25]. Those who were able to keep their consumption at one soft drink or less per week, or were able to decrease to that level, saw a 9–11 pound weight loss [25].

Making a point of emphasizing the detriment of too many sugar-sweetened beverages in any diet is essential, and passing on data-based information to patients on how they can practically impact their diet is extremely useful [30]. Basic messaging like drinking water when they are thirsty, and having a sugar-sweetened beverage for pleasure (rather than thirst), is a sound advice worth repeating at every visit.

Sugar-sweetened beverages (SSBs) can lead to weight gain through their high added-sugar content, low satiety, and an incomplete compensatory reduction in energy intake at subsequent meals after intake of liquid calories. On average, SSBs contain 140–150 calories and 35.0–37.5 g sugar per 12-oz serving. In addition, fructose from any sugar or high fructose-content sugar (HFCS) has been shown to promote the development of visceral adiposity and ectopic fat deposition. [30]

Obesity impacts African Americans in a number of ways including increased coronary heart disease, heart failure, hypertension, stroke, and venous thrombosis. The increased obesity rate drives up type 2 diabetes incidence in both adults and children while also increasing the incidence of fatty liver, obstructive sleep apnea, and degenerative joint disease. As research into the specific ways a patient's eating habits impact them continues, applying the knowledge that already exists to patient-centered diet modification suggestions can add up to a significant impact.

While self-perception in African Americans does blunt some degree of trepidation resulting from obesity, there is still a disproportionate amount of helplessness as it relates to getting practical advice for a sustained benefit.

As primary clinical providers, being able to discuss poor dietary habits and physical inactivity with our patients is critical. But any changes suggested should be incremental. Simply telling a patient to dramatically change their diet and daily lifestyles to something completely foreign to them is a complete waste of time for the patient and the provider. Mapping out planned and incremental suggestions based on the patient's preferences and current lifestyle is essential.

Many providers confuse obesity with gluttony and appear to blame patients for their size and health. In reality, a patient's degree of obesity is a combination of a number of interrelated factors that may or may not be in their control. Success will require a delicate mix of interventions based on treating the patient as the center of the solution. Is the patient's risk for diabetes based on genetics, diet, family cooking patterns, or other factors? Only the patient can tell you, and as the provider, you have a unique opportunity to be granted permission by the patient to make a difference.

Dietary Differences and Ways to Impact Choices

- African Americans eat relatively more chicken and turkey, as well as fish and pork, but less beef than European and Hispanic/Latino American diets.
- African Americans eat relatively more fruit, but fewer vegetables.
- Explain the true impact of frying foods.
- Advise against reusing cooking oil more than twice.
- Dietary AGEs have been suspected to increase diabetes occurrence, cause premature aging, facilitate weight gain, advance carotid stenosis and peripheral artery occlusive disease, worsen kidney disease, and promote the development and progression of heart failure.
- Patient encounters focusing and discussing current dietary habits and physical inactivity is crucial.
- Any change suggestions related to diet and activity levels should be gradual and incremental.
- Dramatic changes from a baseline diet will frequently fail.
- Whenever possible, be specific about the dietary changes you expect.
- Advise a healthy (yet easy) low-fat breakfast daily with a high-fiber food (oatmeal, grits, or fresh fruit).
- African Americans can greatly impact the nutritional value of their meals by simply avoiding frying their foods.
- Quantify your patient's current use of sugar-sweetened beverages, and advise a gradual (yet reasonable) decrease in use.
- An African American woman consumes almost double the sugar-sweetened beverage amounts than European American woman of the same age.
- An African American woman who was able to keep their consumption at one soft drink or less per week, or was able to decrease to that level, saw a sustained 9–11 pound weight loss.
- Be aware that African Americans frequently will be more content at a larger size and may not be aware of the true impact of their size on their future health.

References

1. Standard American Diet. NutritionFacts.org. https://nutritionfacts.org/topics/standard-american-diet/. Accessed 28 May 2019.
2. Commodity Consumption by Population Characteristics. United States Department of Agriculture. Economic Research Service. https://www.ers.usda.gov/data-products/commodity-consumption-by-population-characteristics/. Accessed 28 May 2019.

3. Richardson S, Freedman B, Ellison D, et al. Salt sensitivity: a review with a focus on non-Hispanic blacks and hispanics. J Am Soc Hypertens. 2013;7(2):170–9.
4. African-Americans Combine Tradition with a Multimedia Approach to Shopping. 2016. Retrieved 22 Nov 2018, from https://www.nielsen.com/us/en/insights/news/2016/african-americans-combine-tradition-with-a-multimedia-approach-to-shopping.html.
5. Poti J, Mendez M, Ng S, Popkin B. Is the degree of food processing and convenience linked with the nutritional quality of foods purchased by US households? Am J Clin Nutr. 2015;101(6):1251–62.
6. Sun Y, Liu B, Snetselaar LG, et al. Association of fried food consumption with all cause cardiovascular and cancer mortality: prospective cohort study. BMJ. 2019;364:k5420.
7. Chen H, Wu L, Li Y, Meng J, Lin N, Yang D, et al. Advanced glycation end products increase carbohydrate responsive element binding protein expression and promote cancer cell proliferation. Mol Cell Endocrinol. 2014;395(1–2):69–78.
8. Hegab Z, Gibbons S, Neyses L, Mamas M. Role of advanced glycation end products in cardiovascular disease. World J Cardiol. 2012;4(4):90–102.
9. Park A, Eckert TL, Zaso MJ, et al. Associations between health literacy and health behaviors among urban high school students. J Sch Health. 2017;87(12):885–93.
10. Berkman ND, Sheridan SL, Donahue KE, et al. Low health literacy and health outcomes: an updated systematic review. Ann Intern Med. 2011;155(2):97–107.
11. HDL cholesterol: How to boost your 'good' cholesterol. Mayo Clinic. 2018. https://www.mayoclinic.org/diseases-conditions/high-blood-cholesterol/in-depth/hdl-cholesterol/art-20046388. Accessed 9 June 2019.
12. Cahill L, Pan A, Chiuve S, et al. Fried-food consumption and risk of type 2 diabetes and coronary artery disease: a prospective study in 2 cohorts of US women and men. Am J Clin Nutr. 2014;100(2):667–75.
13. de Souza RJ, Mente A, Maroleanu A, et al. Intake of saturated and trans unsaturated fatty acids and risk of all-cause mortality, cardiovascular disease, and type 2 diabetes: systematic review and meta-analysis of observational studies. BMJ. 2015;351:h3978.
14. Li A, Ha Y, Wang F, Li W, Li Q. Determination of thermally induced trans-fatty acids in soybean oil by attenuated total reflectance Fourier Transform infrared spectroscopy and gas chromatography analysis. J Agric Food Chem. 2012;60(42):10709–13.
15. Affenito SG, Thompson DR, Barton BA, et al. Breakfast consumption by African American and white adolescent girls correlates positively with calcium and fiber intake and negatively with body mass index. J Am Diet Assoc. 2005;105(6):938–45.
16. Rampersaud GC, Pereira MA, Girard BL, et al. Breakfast habits, nutritional status, body weight, and academic performance in children and adolescents. J Am Diet Assoc. 2005;105(5):743–60. https://doi.org/10.1016/j.jada.2005.02.007.
17. Hopkins LC, Sattler M, Anderson Steeves E, et al. Breakfast consumption frequency and its relationships to overall diet quality, using healthy eating index 2010, and body mass index among adolescents in a low-income urban setting. Ecol Food Nutr. 2017;56(4):297–311.
18. O'Neil C, Byrd-Bredbenner C, Hayes D, et al. The role of breakfast in health: definition and criteria for a quality breakfast. J Acad Nutr Diet. 2014;114(12 Suppl):S8–S26.
19. Adolphus K, Lawton CL, Champ CL, Dye L. The effects of breakfast and breakfast composition on cognition in children and adolescents: a systematic review. Adv Nutr. 2016;7:590S–612S.

20. Casazza K, Brown A, Astrup A, et al. Weighing the evidence of common beliefs in obesity research. Crit Rev Food Sci Nutr. 2015;55(14):2014–53.
21. Brown-Riggs C. Nutrition and health disparities: the role of dairy in improving minority health outcomes. Int J Environ Res Public Health. 2015;13(1):28. https://doi.org/10.3390/ijerph13010028.
22. Lactose Intolerance by Ethnicity and Region. ProCon.org. 2018. https://milk.procon.org/view.resource.php?resourceID=000661. Accessed 9 June 2019.
23. Baily RK, Fileti CP, Keith J, et al. Lactose intolerance and health disparities among African Americans and Hispanic Americans: an updated consensus statement. J Natl Med Assoc. 2013;105(2):112–27.
24. Lang SS. Lactose intolerance seems linked to ancestral struggles with harsh climate and cattle diseases, Cornell study finds. 2005. http://news.cornell.edu/stories/2005/06/lactose-intolerance-linked-ancestral-struggles-climate-diseases. Accessed 9 June 2019.
25. Kumanyika SK, Grier SA, Lancaster K, Lassiter V. Impact of sugar-sweetened beverage consumption on black American's health. Robert Wood Johnson Foundation. 2011. https://www.rwjf.org/en/library/research/2011/01/impact-of-sugar-sweetened-beverage-consumption-on-black-american.html. Accessed 9 June 2019.
26. Rosinger A, Herrick K, Gahche J, Park S. Sugar-sweetened beverage consumption among US adults, 2011–2014. NCHS Data Brief. 2017;(270):1–8.
27. Hartman TJ, Haardörfer R, Greene BM, et al. Beverage consumption patterns among overweight and obese African American women. Nutrients. 2017;9(12):pii: E1344.
28. Harris JL, Bargh JA, Brownell KD. Priming effects of television food advertising on eating behavior. Health Psychol. 2009;28:404–13.
29. Grier SA, Kumanyika SK. The context for choice: health implications of targeted food and beverage marketing to African Americans. Am J Public Health. 2008;98:1616–29.
30. Malik VS, Pan A, Willett WC, Hu FB. Sugar-sweetened beverages and weight gain in children and adults: a systematic review and meta-analysis. Am J Clin Nutr. 2013;98(4):1084–102.

Connecting with Stories: Improving Patient Adherence and Compliance

14

The African American tradition extends deeply into African tribal customs. The telling of stories to convey knowledge and experience is as old as time [1, 2]. For the African people, the oral tradition defined their cultural heritage. The spoken word was how traditions, folktales, histories, and religious convictions were passed from one generation to the next [2]. Family histories and stories were learned, memorized, and recounted as a way to remember the past, and in many parts of Africa, that tradition continues to this day. If the story did not evoke an emotion, be it laughter, agreement, concern, or some other feeling, the story was lost to the listener. So the storyteller and their proper preparation were critical to the success of the story.

In general, stories are easier to remember than facts. Stories come with a context and details meant to include the listener. Because stories are told with more than just words, the listener remembers the details and the emotions. This is in sharp contrast to histories which are merely an account of events. Clinicians deal in histories all the time.

> The patient was cutting his grass when he began to have chest pain, sat down, and then called 911.

We've been trained to listen to the history, pull out key elements, ask relevant questions, and then come up with helpful recommendations. Stories, or narratives, require forethought, are usually better organized, and have a moral and an intended outcome in the listener. Many patients with viral upper respiratory infections come to clinicians with "stories" designed to prompt a desired outcome: prescribed antibiotics. They know that certain elements of their story will trigger the antibiotic button in us and the absence of those triggers will not. By embellishing their history into a story, patients will frequently get what they want.

© Springer Nature Switzerland AG 2020
G. L. Hall, *Patient-Centered Clinical Care for African Americans*,
https://doi.org/10.1007/978-3-030-26418-5_14

If a story can be told to manipulate trained clinicians into action, surely we can build our arsenal of accurate, motivational narratives to tell and inspire our patients.

JoAnne Banks-Wallace believed stories and storytelling were also a cornerstone of qualitative research [2]:

> Story creation and storytelling enable us to give unique expression to our experiences, the wisdom gleaned through living, and truths passed on from generation to generation. Storytelling steeped in oral traditions provides unique opportunities to contribute to the development and testing of theories or interventions while promoting the health of study participants. [2]

In African history, the storytellers played a significant role as the human voice, and presentation style was critical to the successful communication of the details and sentiment of a story. Stories were organized, rehearsed, and presented as a way to perpetuate tribal histories, herbal medicine ingredients, and healing techniques through a conduit story that, if misremembered, would impact not just one, but all subsequent generations.

14.1 Storytelling Influences Start Early

This predilection for stories starts early in the African American culture, and educators have found reliable and persistent differences in the learning and advancement of African American children and their ability to tell and interpret a story [3, 4]. African American children tell stories that are "vivid, elaborate, and rich in imagery" says Nicole Gardner-Neblett from the University of North Carolina's Frank Porter Graham Child Development Institute. She found distinct differences in how early storytelling skills in African American children impacted later literacy. Dr. Gardner-Neblett states:

> The strong storytelling skills of African-American children may stem from the cultural and historic influences that have fostered a preference for orality among African Americans. [3]

By considering African American's "preference for orality" and the imagery and mastery of stories as a way to connect and learn, we clinicians will merely be taking a path of least resistance when it comes to connecting with the many patients that appreciate stories.

Abject data, like most of the information we give our patients, is decontextualized from the standpoint of our listeners. We have spent years learning basic sciences and have progressed to super-specialized clinicians. When explaining the impact of any particular medical intervention, we speak from a very learned context, one that is dramatically distant from most of our patients. Taking the time and energy to translate that information into actionable stories will be an impactful and efficient use of our time. Once well-crafted contextualized stories are developed, they can be individually refined and used repeatedly on countless patients.

14.2   Marketing for Good Health

Salesmen and marketers have touted the importance of using stories to improve a brand, sell a product, inspire interest, and advance long-term product loyalty. In medicine, the goals for our patients are strikingly similar. We want to inspire them to understand their disorder and make the appropriate changes in their lifestyle. We need to motivate them to take their medications regularly, modify their diet, and increase their exercise in a way that is stimulating and memorable.

By using a storytelling approach, we can help our patients better internalize their medical problem, see where they are impacting it negatively, and then inspire them to make the appropriate changes that will have a lasting positive impression.

Interviews of successful physicians across racial populations find that storytelling is a valuable and integral part of educating patients about the merit of a clinical intervention [5]. Successful physicians tell stories all the time. These physicians, with high patient satisfaction scores, frequently tell relatable stories and personal disclosures about their family and friends as a way to connect with their patients.

Many successful physicians report that they "stumbled" onto stories as a tactic to help them convince a skeptical patient and, after seeing early and consistent success, incorporated the telling of stories into their daily routine. Encouraging physicians to tell stories is not new. John Steiner wrote about the use of stories in clinical settings and proposed many of the same components emphasized in marketing: getting the customer's point of view through a clinical interrogation and then telling a good story based on a narrative competence [6].

Kenneth Calman compared stories to viruses:

> It is suggested that behavior can change because of ideas transmitted, often in the form of stories from one person to another. Such a mechanism may involve transmids (transmitted ideas). The analogy can be developed further, in that such contagion depends on virulence, and on the resistance of the listener. Like micro-organisms, some ideas are dangerous. [5]

Patients will frequently be told a story by a neighbor or friend that is completely counterproductive. A patient hobbling on a knee that needs replacement will reject the suggestion because of a horrific story of a bad outcome. Much of the success of herbs and home remedies rely on stories of healing.

Physicians have a long history of submitting interesting "case reports" to journals and colleagues as a way to stimulate discussion, gather input, and generally form the foundation for future research. These accounts of unusual clinical outcomes are merely well-crafted stories. Steiner wrote:

> Clinical stories are used in many ways: to inform, to share, to inspire, to educate, and to persuade. Physicians constantly use the stories they hear to inform decisions and actions that directly affect the patient subject. [6]

Professional marketers are specifically instructed to tell stories as an early approach to establish trust and allegiance [7]. There are countless articles and books on marketing stories as a way to sell almost anything. In marketing, the telling of stories as a way to "connect" to the customer is fully accepted as the only true path to success. A good story contains these five components:

1. A subject or hero
2. A goal
3. A conflict or obstacle
4. A mentor
5. A moral

When applying these marketing elements to a clinical approach to storytelling, we see a natural fit. The *hero* is *always* the patient or, more often, a surrogate for the patient, someone "just like the patient" who had similar challenges and overcame them.

The *goal* is the "transformation" that the hero is seeking: good health, more energy, longer life, better endurance, etc. It is critical that clinicians fully elucidate and understand our hero/patient's goal. In hypertension, it usually is *not* controlled blood pressure (that is the clinician's goal). Their goal is more likely to "feel healthier," as evidenced by more energy, stamina, fewer discomforts, and/or the absence of life-threatening events (heart attacks and strokes).

The *obstacles* in our story may be internal or external in origin. With most of our stories dealing with internal motivational obstacles that must be overcome to reach a healthy steady state, it is the obstacles that make the story motivational.

The clinician is the *mentor*, and rightfully so. We have the knowledge, training, and expertise to help the subject overcome health obstacles. If the patient is Luke Skywalker, then the physician is Obi-Wan Kenobi. We are the wise mentors who can provide essential information and tools that allow the hero subject to attain their goal.

And finally, marketers stress that the *moral* of any story should be clear and concise. The patient was less than what they should have been. While their goal was to have a transformation, there were obstacles in the form of motivation, understanding, and trust. Ultimately these barriers were overcome and a remarkable and honest *truth* evolved.

Adapting this generally accepted model for motivational clinical stories has wide-ranging potential for better communication, understanding, compliance, and improved outcomes. Researchers are currently investigating the impact of storytelling on a host of problems including smoking cessation [8] at a VA hospital in Massachusetts, hypertension [9] control by using successful personal narratives in a theater setting, a compilation of patient-reported storytelling of their success with smoking cessation, and much more. As the power of storytelling and its relation to African American influence improves, the ways to apply stories in pursuit of better health will grow.

While these components of a story are popularly linked to marketing approaches, Jerome Bruner, noted psychologist, author, and law professor from Harvard, wrote that "it is no surprise that story is the coin and currency of culture." In his book, *Making Stories: Law, Literature, Life*, Bruner examines the usefulness of stories as they relate to business strategies, legal success with judges and juries, and their application in effective writing [10].

Bruner emphasized that the key component of a story is the obstacle... "For there to be a story something unforeseen must happen. There is an unexpected turn of events, a peripeteia as Aristotle said" [10]. In our clinical world, the peripeteia is the medical intervention, because without its presence, the patient's life course was headed in a dire direction. The uncontrolled hypertension was spiraling toward a fatal stroke or heart attack. The unbridled smoking was feeding cancerous cells in their infancy. And then we, the clinicians, arrive with life-saving advice.

Bruner also stressed that the cultural perspective of the narrator and the subject must be considered as culture explains both the origin of the problem as well as the key to the solution. Trying to convince a person that comes from a family where everyone smokes is a greater challenge due to their cultural affirmation that smoking is "okay." Getting a thorough family history that shows premature death from smoking-related illnesses and approaching the patient with the long-livers in their family who did not smoke uses a logical "you-gave-me-the-history" evidence-based argument that few could refute.

Finally, Bruner stressed that the story is bound by its verisimilitude (and yes I had to look that word up too). Culture's "myths and its folktales, its dramas and its pageants memorialize both its norms and notable violations of them" [10]. Verisimilitude means the story must "ring true" to the listener, or the impact will be lost. Therefore, the culture and history of the listener must be artfully embedded into the story respectfully and with regard for the cultural perspectives assigned to the narrator by the listener. This explains why reformed alcoholics are the best mentors and teachers for current alcoholics. They both have a common historical perspective and a number of stories to tell to motivate action. Someone who never drank alcohol comes with little perspective to convince others … unless they have a really good story.

14.3   The Patient's Perspective

"I don't want medicine … is there a vitamin I can take?"
I have frequently told my patients to not discriminate against the medications I prescribe "just because they've been proven to work." After the FDA has approved a medication for use and demonstrated that it works across a population, it has to be monitored and regulated, whether prescription or over-the-counter. It seems that as soon as a medication requires a prescription, many of my patients want to avoid it. Somehow the medication has become tainted, and rather than be energetic about the proven prospects for a longer life and good health, they become depressed and bemoan the fact that they have to take a medication for "the rest of their life." This reaction, however dysfunctional, is based on a learned and trained response that we clinicians taught them.

When presented with elevated blood pressure in African Americans, our response is casual and typical. After all, the vast majority of African Americans we see in the medical environment have hypertension, as do almost half of all African Americans. Hypertension is so commonplace in African Americans that we do not take the time to frame the problem properly, explain the far-reaching implications, or fully praise the miraculous potential of antihypertensive medications.

Studies have repeatedly shown that controlled blood pressure increases energy and stamina, reduces fatigue, and bolsters well-being [11, 12]. In addition, hypertensive therapy saves a resounding number of lives and dramatically decreases cardiovascular events including heart attack, stroke, and congestive heart failure [11, 12]. What this data confirms across racial populations is even more impactful in African Americans who have a disproportionate percentage with these deadly diseases.

The reality of hypertension is it does progressive damage to the circulatory system, and the proper functioning of the circulatory system is essential to the basic functions of both major and minor organs. The medical establishment frequently says that hypertension is asymptomatic … the silent killer, but studies have confirmed that it actually negatively impacts a patient's quality of life [13]. Put simply, there are symptoms in untreated hypertension that improve after therapy.

In striking contrast, the stories patients typically have heard about blood pressure medications are all sad. "They make you have to go to the bathroom all the time."

"They kill an erection." "They make you tired." These narratives drain all of the excitement and motivation from patients. Rather than thinking of the prospect of living a longer, healthier life, they are now burdened with feeling that they will be taking a pill for the rest of their life.

In medicine, our usual approach is one of lecturing. Since we know the truth about what ails our patients, we simply present our solution … take it or leave it. Unfortunately, many African Americans will "leave it." Because of the fundamental lack of trust for the medical establishment that many African Americans feel, just giving out "the facts" of our ailment is far from adequate. We need to take the time to formulate an inspirational story that is patient centered and diagnostically appropriate.

Interviewing the patient to elicit their exercise tolerance, baseline energy levels, and activities of daily living, and then offering an opportunity to improve their function, sheds an entirely new light on antihypertensive therapy. By going one step further and determining the patient's emotional wants (feeling better) versus their simple needs (lowering blood pressure), and then aiming therapeutic goals and future discussions at their wants rather than the needs, clinicians can positively impact overall compliance and satisfaction.

14.4 Hypertension and Diabetes Examples

When telling the story about hypertension,
… talk about the stress that high blood pressure places on arteries and veins throughout their body … day in and day out … the wearing down of the basic foundations of their systems. The unrelenting strain that their vessels see as they try to stay intact and properly deliver organ-saving oxygen and nutrients to their muscles, brain, heart, liver, bone marrow, and much more. The literal abuse of their bodies running on overdrive all the time, yet yearning for relief. It's no wonder there is fatigue, irritation, anxiety, inefficiency, and sporadic malfunctions in patients with hypertension.

By starting clinically proven medications for blood pressure, we restore normal blood and vessel function, boost endurance, and fortify the bodies' normal performance. In addition to safely and effectively improving everyday function, these medications will extend life through dramatically decreased stroke, heart attack, and kidney failure.

After starting antihypertension medications, some patients feel a little fatigued. If they do, it is because their body has been strained for an extended period of time and is finally able (and needs) to rest. Calling the initial physiological response to finally feeling a normal blood pressure, a medication side effect, is wholly inaccurate and misleading. The body is finally, after years of progressive unrelenting strain, seeing normality … give it a chance to recover and rest. Be thankful that no permanent damage was done in overdrive. Let the body recover.

Needless to say, every story does not fit every person. The interview that elicits the details of our patient's emotional wants will drive the content of each story. It is also important to use what author Richard Bayan calls "Words that Sell" [14]. These are time-tested words that paint a positive picture. Marketers know and agree that certain words have more energy, are more inspiring, and can move more people into action. Purposely adding these words to your stories for health will improve communication and help compliance.

When telling the story about diabetes,

… talk about how African Americans are disproportionately impacted with diabetes being 80 percent more likely to be diagnosed initially, four times more likely to be diagnosed with kidney disease leading to dialysis, and 3.5 times more likely to have a leg amputation. African Americans are twice as likely to die from diabetes than European Americans [15].

Patients with uncontrolled diabetes lead to poor quality lives for a number of reasons. In addition to the inefficient processing of sugars in the blood, the elevated sugars have a devastating impact on health in a number of ways. Based on the list below, determine which are affected in your patient.

- *The increased sugar impairs kidney function which causes increased water loss through excessive urination … both day and night … leading to dehydration.*
- *Kidney function: the elevated glucose impacts the body's ability to filter water.*
- *Poor digestion: because of dehydration and nerve damage, diabetes impacts the enjoyment and digestion of food.*
- *High blood glucose levels contribute to the formation of fatty deposits in blood vessel walls that can restrict blood flow and increase the risk of hardening of the blood vessels.*
- *The lack of blood flow causes decreased exercise tolerance, walking distances, and wound healing.*
- *Diabetes causes changes in the skin with drying and cracking, increased boils, ulcers, and calluses.*
- *Diabetes causes damage to the nerves which can affect the perception of heat, cold, and pain and is making you more susceptible to accidental injury.*
- *Swollen, leaky blood vessels in the eye (diabetic retinopathy) can damage your vision and even lead to blindness.*
- *People with diabetes tend to develop cataracts at an earlier age.*

Your goal will be to fix whichever problems (obvious and subtle) you find are most negatively impacting the patient. But also try to quantify how negatively impacted is their overall quality of life, emphasizing the background damage occurring that is not among their complaints, but present nonetheless.

How often are tasks you want to complete interrupted by the need to urinate? How has your perception of heat or cold changed? You can clearly see that your quality of life is a mere fraction of what it was?

Metformin takes the most natural approach to lowering your elevated blood sugars by having your body naturally absorb the excess sugar. It has the added benefit that if you take in food that worsens the diabetes, your body will quickly flush it out of your system. All of the medicines for diabetes have been clinically tested and proven to be safe and effective. In no time, you will feel invigorated and energized, while your metabolism and immune system are enhanced.

14.5 Worldview = Culture

Marketers talk about approaching potential customers by using their "worldview." Market and branding author Jeff Korhan defines a worldview as "a philosophy or set of values through which people interpret and interact with the world" [16].

The approach to convincing anyone of anything involves discerning their worldview and then framing the approach appropriately, a marketer would say. A person's cultural history is just another term for worldview … how the person, or patient, sees things. If we are to be successful in convincing our patients of anything, we need to understand their life's perspective, their worldview … their culture.

By looking at clinicians' perspective for why African Americans do or do not do anything, the reason is embedded in their culture. When clinicians look at their own clinical behavior and outcomes, the explanations for their successes and failures are embedded in their culture as well. The "value" that clinicians place on a distinguished gentleman with chest pain versus a homeless alcoholic smoker with chest pain is dramatically different, and clinical outcome data confirm it consistently [17, 18]. The decreased value, whether conscious or subconscious, drives the speed, number, and quality of the subsequent interventions.

Objective protocols for serious presentations, like angina, have dramatically decreased disparities in outcomes for chest pain in the emergency department [19]. The subjective "clinical calls" that used to be made when an individual presented with chest pain resulted in differences in myocardial infarction outcomes based on race and sex. By removing the clinicians' personal cultural perspective from the equation, health disparities shrunk.

But removing the clinician's cultural perspective from the encounter essentially removes the clinician, which needless to say, also results in poor clinical outcomes. The obvious answer is to open the clinicians' perception to other worldviews, or cultural perspectives, so that they can consider how their culture colors the clinical picture at hand.

Cultural competence and patient-centered care are really pseudonyms for knowing a patient's worldview before advancing or framing an approach to their care. We currently are telling patients what they should do and in many ways are trying to sell a person something they do not want. Instead, we need to understand their cultural view and then tailor our approach to be complementary. Connect with your patients by understanding their personal culture, and then adapt your educational approach accordingly.

Connecting with Stories
- By using a storytelling approach, we can help our patients better internalize their medical problems and help them make the appropriate changes.
- A good story has these five components:

  1. A subject or hero
  2. A goal
  3. A conflict or obstacle
  4. A mentor
  5. A moral

- To be successful in convincing our patients, we need to understand their life's perspective (their culture).

References

1. Alvarez. African story telling. 2014. https://prezi.com/uq3pxvnigfoq/african-story-telling/. Accessed 9 June 2019.
2. Banks-Wallace J. Talk that talk: storytelling and analysis rooted in African American oral tradition. Qual Health Res. 2002;12(3):410–26.
3. Gardner-Neblett N. Why storytelling skills matter for African-American kids. 2018. Retrieved November 22, 2018, from https://theconversation.com/why-storytelling-skills-matter-for-african-american-kids-46844.

4. Champion T. Understanding storytelling among African American children. n.d. Retrieved November 22, 2018, from https://books.google.com/books?hl=en&lr=&id=5XuRAgAAQBA J&oi=fnd&pg=PP1&dq=tempiichampionbook&ots=u6FexFy8Kh&sig=nUUvxu4HI6vjdjbcx SVkJTA9OqM#v=onepage&q=tempii champion book&f=false.

5. Calman K. A study of storytelling, humour and learning in medicine. Clin Med (Lond). 2001;1(3):227–9.

6. Steiner JF. The use of stories in clinical research and health policy. JAMA. 2005;294(22):2901. https://doi.org/10.1001/jama.294.22.2901.

7. Godin S. All marketers are liars (Tell Stories). The underground classic that explains how marketing really works – and why authenticity is the best marketing of all. New York: Portfolio; 2012.

8. Cherrington A, Williams J, Foster P. Narratives to enhance smoking cessation interventions among African-American smokers, the ACCE project. BMC Res Notes. 2015;8(1):567. https://doi.org/10.1186/s13104-015-1513-1.

9. Fix G, Houston T, Barker A, et al. A novel process for integrating patient stories into patient education interventions: incorporating lessons from theater arts. Patient Educ Couns. 2012;88(3):455–9.

10. Bruner JS. Making stories: law, literature, life. Cambridge, MA: Harvard University Press; 2003.

11. Fryar CD, Ostchega Y, Hales CM, et al. Hypertension prevalence and control among adults: United States, 2015–2016. NCHS Data Brief. 2017;(289):1–8.

12. Zhang Y, Moran AE. Trends in the prevalence, awareness, treatment, and control of hypertension among young adults in the United States, 1999–2014. Hypertension. 2017;70(4):736–42.

13. Hypertension (normal Vs. high blood pressure). n.d. Retrieved November 22, 2018, from https://my.clevelandclinic.org/health/diseases/4314-hypertension-high-blood-pressure.

14. Bayan R. Words that sell. 2nd ed. New York: McGraw-Hill Education; 2006.

15. Office of Minority Health. n.d. Retrieved November 22, 2018, from https://minorityhealth.hhs. gov/omh/browse.aspx?lvl=4&lvlid=18.

16. Korhan J. Marketing to the worldview of your customers – Jeff Korhan. 2014. Retrieved November 22, 2018, from http://www.jeffkorhan.com/2014/06/marketing-to-worldview-your-customers.html.

17. Ghail JK, Cooper RS, Kowatly I, Liao Y. Delay between onset of chest pain and arrival to the coronary care unit among minority and disadvantaged patients. J Natl Med Assoc. 1993;85(3):180–4.

18. Pawlik TM, Olver IN, Storm CD, Rodriguez MA. Can physicians refuse treatment to patients who smoke? J Oncol Pract. 2009;5(5):250–1.

19. 2015 National Healthcare Quality and Disparities Report Chartbook on Health Care for Blacks. Rockville: Agency for Healthcare Research and Quality; 2016. AHRQ Pub. No 16-0015-1-EF.

An "Oath" and a Responsibility

15

I swear to fulfill, to the best of my ability and judgment, this covenant:

I will respect the hard-won scientific gains of those physicians in whose steps I walk, and gladly share such knowledge as is mine with those who are to follow.

I will apply, for the benefit of the sick, all measures which are required, avoiding those twin traps of overtreatment and therapeutic nihilism.

I will remember that there is art to medicine as well as science, and that warmth, sympathy, and understanding may outweigh the surgeon's knife or the chemist's drug.

I will not be ashamed to say " I know not," nor will I fail to call in my colleagues when the skills of another are needed for a patient's recovery.

I will respect the privacy of my patients, for their problems are not disclosed to me that the world may know. Most especially must I tread with care in matters of life and death. Above all, I must not play at God.

I will remember that I do not treat a fever chart, a cancerous growth, but a sick human being, whose illness may affect the person's family and economic stability. My responsibility includes these related problems, if I am to care adequately for the sick.

© Springer Nature Switzerland AG 2020

G. L. Hall, *Patient-Centered Clinical Care for African Americans*,

https://doi.org/10.1007/978-3-030-26418-5_15

I will prevent disease whenever I can but I will always look for a path to a cure for all diseases.

I will remember that I remain a member of society, with special obligations to all my fellow human beings, those sound of mind and body as well as the infirm.

If I do not violate this oath, may I enjoy life and art, respected while I live and remembered with affection thereafter. May I always act so as to preserve the finest traditions of my calling and may I long experience the joy of healing those who seek my help.

(This "modern version" of the Hippocratic Oath was written in 1964 by Louis Lasagna, Dean of the School of Medicine at Tufts University.)

The honor and responsibilities of being a clinical provider are best characterized by the centuries-old Hippocratic Oath. Written as a welcoming to new physicians to medical practice, updated versions of this Greek medical text are mainstays at medical graduations across the world [1–4].

While recited at the end of a long and grueling educational process, many repeat the oath without much thought or reflection. But the content of the oath sets the stage for a very rewarding and successful clinical practice, a common thread of decency, humility, respect, and responsibility course through the passages. The fact that this "oath" in its various translations has lasted over 2000 years is a testament to the foundational truths it dictates.

Not adhering to these tenets has resulted in many of the deficiencies and disparities we see in modern medicine. Avoiding "therapeutic nihilism" in its many forms including defensive medicine and therapies for profit all represents the downsides of clinical care. The lack of respect for privacy in the Tuskegee Syphilis Study resounds as one of the many incredible injustices that were overseen by physicians. And the "special obligations" providers have to fellow human beings must transgress political parties, sexual orientations, and other differences that make humans human. Re-centering our care to best treat a specific population by "all measures which are required" is an obligation by oath, as well as a recipe for a successful clinical practice.

The oath also describes our added responsibilities that include "the person's family and economic stability." While some providers consider these as "outside" of their control, the presumption is to merely "consider" these modifiers of health and include them in your treatment discussion and plan. Consider a patient's spouses' ability to influence their diet and include them in discussions related to nutrition. Consider the patient's ability to travel to consultants or for studies, and discuss what needs to take place in order for there to be a successful follow-through.

> The major attributes of Hippocratic morality can be summarized as follows: the first characteristic is that Hippocratic medicine is individualistic, that is, the physician acts always in the best interest of the patient, which implies the moral obligation of beneficent and consequently nonmaleficent. The aim of any medical procedure is the good of the patient independently of other factors, such as the ability to pay or the background of the patient. [4]

None of these doctrines are new, and they essentially amount to basic common sense. We have sacred responsibilities that are almost as old as time itself, and while perspectives vary, with all of the advancements and technologies at our disposal, the basic ethics of the Hippocratic Oath have not changed.

The "Florence Nightingale Pledge" developed in 1893 for nurses has the same ethical tone and central themes [5]:

> I solemnly pledge myself before God and in the presence of this assembly, to pass my life in purity and to practice my profession faithfully. I will abstain from whatever is deleterious and mischievous, and will not take or knowingly administer any harmful drug. I will do all in my power to maintain and elevate the standard of my profession, and will hold in confidence all personal matters committed to my keeping and all family affairs coming to my knowledge in the practice of my calling. With loyalty will I endeavor to aid the physician, in his work, and devote myself to the welfare of those committed to my care. [5]

15.1 Foundations of Medical Ethics

From an ethics standpoint, the four basic principles of medical ethics developed by Beauchamp and Childress also nicely describe the foundations of good clinical care [6]:

- *Beneficence* describes the concept of acting for the patient's good.
- *Nonmaleficence* describes the concept of doing no harm.
- *Autonomy* conveys the idea that each patient has a right to voice his or her own values and choices about care.
- *Justice* expresses the idea that healthcare resources should be equitably distributed among patients and that patients should be treated fairly.

These four foundations of medical ethics are also in line with health equity teachings. By following prescriptions and recommendations tailored for African American outcomes, we act for the "patient's good," and by appropriately changing our care to align with published research that shows inferior outcomes, we do less harm. Building trust with our patients involves, among other things, identifying with their values and priorities. And finally, true justice in medicine is personified by every patient having access to medical care and a choice when decisions are made about their life.

It is certainly not unusual for providers to be unaware of nuances that apply to isolated special populations. Primary care providers are occasionally presented with patients with Down's syndrome or HIV and may not be the best authority on their care due to a very low volume presenting to their practice. When presented with a patient with a unique clinical demographic, providers will usually brush up quickly on the topic and then refer to a specialist for more definitive interventions. When we repeatedly see the same presentations or unique populations, we slowly become authorities in the nuances of care in that population.

There is no question that many providers "anecdotally" saw that ACE inhibitors were inferior to calcium channel blockers when trying to reach blood pressure goals in African Americans. Oncologists saw more aggressive presentations of breast and prostate cancer in African Americans as well. Many of these clinical observations led to the research that verified their suspicions. Clinicians then incorporate those differences into their clinical practice for the better of their patient population. Somehow incorporating this nuanced care for African Americans' benefit has eluded some clinicians' threshold of notice, and numerous research outcomes continue to confirm this. By recognizing these important differences and applying them appropriately, everyone wins.

15.2   Misunderstandings

It is also important to note that some of the poor outcomes seen in African Americans result from misguided assumptions and misunderstandings that ultimately undermine a clinicians' best intentions when trying to provide quality care. Health literacy may be a stronger predictor of personal health than age, employment status, education level, race, or income. While a student's literacy is frequently tied to their teacher's ability to teach, a patient's health literacy is frequently proportional to their clinician's ability to communicate the nuances of medical care in ways that their patients can understand. For example, patient education and health literacy were shown to greatly improve the nutrient quality of many patients' diet, a study by Kuczmarski and colleagues at the University of Delaware determined [7]. Health literacy leads to improved patient self-management support in chronic diseases like diabetes, heart failure, and hypertension and is critical to improving long-term quality outcomes [8–13].

Some degree of poor compliance with medications in African Americans can be attributed to cultural misunderstandings of the known causes of many conditions. A clinician's knowledge of these common misperceptions can greatly facilitate provider-patient conversations and allow for much more efficient visits and productive outcomes. Beliefs that are generationally embedded in a culture will take repetition and trust-building during clinical visits to dispel.

Gbenga Ogedegbe and colleagues at Columbia University looked at prevalent African American beliefs of the causes and treatments for common conditions [14]. For example, a great number confirm that African Americans attribute "stress" to many ailments including hypertension, stroke, myocardial infarctions, and more [15–17]. While some research has suggested that "stress" leads to increased cortisol which worsens obesity, hypertension, kidney failure, and others, patients pin their cure for the stress-induced condition on becoming "stress-free." Achieving the nirvana of becoming stress-free has eluded African Americans, and everyone else, since the beginning of time. When looking at the perceived best treatment for hypertension, the knowledge/literacy disconnect persists. A full 92% of respondents reported that hypertension was "best" treated with garlic, herbs, and vitamins, while physician-prescribed medicines ranked third. The disconnect driving health literacy issues greatly impact compliance and acceptance of advice [18].

Causes of hypertension according to African American focus groups [9]:
1. Stress (100% of groups interviewed)
2. Heredity (83%)
3. Consumption of pork (67%)
4. Salt intake (67%)
5. Excessive use of alcohol (67%)
6. Overweight (67%)
7. Evil spirits (42%)

The most commonly perceived treatments for hypertension according to African American focus groups included [9]:
1. Garlic (92% of groups)
2. Herbs/vitamins (92%)
3. Physician-prescribed medications (83%)
4. Vinegar (75%)
5. Diet or weight loss (67%)

15.3   Recognizing and Correcting Barriers to Good Care

Researchers at the Cleveland Clinic developed a framework for looking at compliance in patients and categorized four types of barriers [18]:

1. Patient-specific barriers
2. Medication-specific barriers
3. Disease-specific barriers
4. Logistical barriers

Patient-specific barriers   included (1) forgetfulness; (2) beliefs that medications were associated with impotence or drug dependence/addiction or are not needed when one feels well; and (3) attitudes such as denial or feelings that medications are not needed if there is no family history of hypertension and that medications are associated with other poor outcomes such as development of kidney disease or diabetes mellitus, as well as being required to take medications for the rest of one's life.

Medication-specific barriers   included side effects such as allergies, dizziness, headaches, and loss of sexual drive or desire.

Disease-specific barriers   included the absence of symptoms, which was interpreted as implying the lack of need for treatment.

Logistical barriers   included the burden of filling prescriptions, making office visits, having to use the restroom while away from home, and having to carry extra medications to avoid missing a dose [18].

When discussing poor compliance with medications, try to categorize the patient's barriers to taking the medication. If it is forgetfulness, examine their routine and try to develop a better approach. Ashish Atreja and colleagues wrote about ways to improve compliance and grouped the interventions into categories that could be remembered by the mnemonic "SIMPLE" [18]:

- Simplify the regimen.
- Impart knowledge.
- Modify beliefs.
- Provider communication is ineffective.
- Leave the bias.
- Evaluate adherence.

Many patients believe that their hypertension medications need to be taken with food and will carry their pills around with them "until they eat." Amlodipine and hydrochlorothiazide are usually well tolerated on an empty stomach. If the patient bushes their teeth daily, have them associate the taking of medication with teeth brushing instead of food. A large percentage of African Americans never eat breakfast [19]. Have the patient make that one modification and re-evaluate their adherence at their next visit.

Emmanuel Fai and colleagues looked at attitudes of patients and their intention to stay on diabetes medications [20]:

> The findings suggest that attitudes, intentions and perceived behavioral control predict adherence to the use of oral antihyperglycemic regimens in African Americans. In addition, the findings suggest that individuals who perceive taking their type 2 diabetes medications as easy and those with a positive perception about taking their type 2 diabetes medications have high adherence to the use of oral antihyperglycemic regimens. [20]

The attitude and intention of African American patients were shown to be directly correlated with improved compliance. Seeing the task as "easy" greatly improved outcomes. Explaining the rationale and simple mechanism of action for a particular medicine will greatly improve outcomes both individually and across a population [21].

15.4   Small Improvements Within a Population Can Yield Impressive Gains

The effects of a positive impact in the health of African Americans can have wide-ranging and highly sustainable benefits. For example, Hardy and colleagues in the *Journal of the American Heart Association* used multivariate linear regression to estimate benefit from a 1 mm Hg lowering of blood pressure and a 10% proportional reduction in the hypertensive aware, untreated, and uncontrolled [22]. They found that very modest decreases in blood pressure can have dramatic improvements in outcomes particularly in African Americans, likely because there is much more disease to prevent. If all patients did just a little bit better, dramatic improvements in outcomes can be expected. For example, taking the reported 33% of African Americans currently on ACE inhibitors for monotherapy of hypertension and shifting them to a more efficacious medication will undoubtedly save lives.

Lowering the HbA1c has been proven to improve outcomes across populations including decreased heart failure [23], lower extremity amputations [24], and other benefits. With African Americans having a higher incidence of diabetes, achieving better glycemic control will substantially decrease disease burden.

Steven Woolf and colleagues wrote about "the health impact of resolving racial disparities" by analyzing mortality data [25]:

> The US health system spends far more on the "technology" of care (e.g., drugs, devices) than on achieving equity in its delivery. For 1991 to 2000, we contrasted the number of lives saved by medical advances with the number of deaths attributable to excess mortality among African Americans. Medical advances averted 176,633 deaths, but equalizing the mortality rates of Whites and African Americans would have averted 886,202 deaths. Achieving equity may do more for health than perfecting the technology of care. [25]

By determining that five deaths could be avoided for every life saved by medical advances, Woolf put the country's healthcare priorities into perspective. By saving lives with what we know already, we can advance as a society.

Looking at life expectancy, African Americans have made great improvements over the last 50 years in large part due to improved medical care. In short, our efforts thus far have produced significant benefit. In 1960 the average life expectancy of African Americans was 63.6 years, while European Americans' lifespan was 70.6 years [26]. Most recent data shows a gain of 11 years (74.8) for African Americans versus just under 8 years for European Americans (78.5 years). These improvements came at the hand of clinicians across the country who cared enough to improve access to hospitals, nursing facilities, physician practices, and other healthcare entities. While access is still an issue in some places in the United States, our next step is to identify clinical differences and through research and reviewed quality outcomes apply nuanced care to this special population. Figure 15.1 shows a significantly decreased death rate for African Americans over a 16-year span [27].

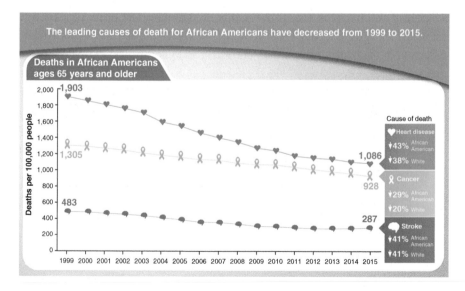

Fig. 15.1 The leading causes of death for African Americans have decreased from 1999 to 2015. https://www.cdc.gov/vitalsigns/aahealth/index.html

Despite the numerous differences described in the preceding chapters, there are far more clinical treatment similarities between African Americans and the other racial groups. Infections, orthopedics, muscle disorders, head and neck pathologies, and much more generally have very similar clinical prevalence, approaches to therapy, and outcomes, when compared with a racial or ethnic eye.

But African Americans still carry the unique and unenviable distinction of being the population in America that has the worst clinical outcomes. Finding ways to reverse this heavy burden should be a priority of every clinician that sees African American patients.

As individual providers, attempting to change society's approach to race and ethnicity is a daunting task, but adjusting our care for patient's sitting in front of us, and asking for our help, is completely within our capacity and responsibility. While no clinician intentionally provides poor medical care, giving good care to all patients in a practice requires thoughtful alacrity. Parents frequently find that raising multiple children in one household successfully requires an array of approaches depending on the child—what worked for one may completely fail another. Using the same approach with all patients will also show variable outcomes.

Quality providers also recognize the "differences" in patients and adjust their approach and care accordingly. Recognizing these differences and applying validated nuanced approaches in care is the pure and simple purpose of this text.

The age-old Hippocratic Oath ends with:

> If I do not violate this oath, may I enjoy life and art, respected while I live and remembered with affection thereafter. May I always act so as to preserve the finest traditions of my calling and may I long experience the joy of healing those who seek my help.

An "Oath" and a Responsibility
- Recognizing the important differences that exist among populations and applying them appropriately ensures quality patient care for everyone.
- The disconnect driving health literacy issues greatly impact compliance and acceptance of advice.
- African Americans have the worst overall clinical outcomes. Reducing this disparity should be the priority of every clinician that sees African American patients.
- Four basic principles of medical ethics:
  - *Beneficence* describes the concept of acting for the patient's good.
  - *Nonmaleficence* describes the concept of doing no harm.
  - *Autonomy* conveys the idea that each patient has a right to voice his or her own values and choices about care.
  - *Justice* expresses the idea that healthcare resources should be equitably distributed among patients and that patients should be treated fairly.

- Some poor outcomes seen in African Americans result from misguided assumptions and misunderstandings on the patient's part. Gaining insight into some of the more common misconceptions can be beneficial.
- African Americans attribute "stress" to many ailments including hypertension, stroke, myocardial infarctions, and more.
- Improve patient compliance by using the mnemonic "SIMPLE":
  - *S*implify the regimen.
  - *I*mpart knowledge.
  - *M*odify beliefs.
  - *P*rovider communication is ineffective.
  - *L*eave the bias.
  - *E*valuate adherence.
- Modest decreases in blood pressure can have dramatic improvements in outcomes particularly in African Americans.
- African Americans have made great improvements over the last 50 years with an 11-year increase in life expectancy.

References

1. Clark S. The impact of the Hippocratic Oath in 2018: the conflict of the ideal of the physician, the knowledgeable humanitarian, versus the corporate medical allegiance to financial models contributes to burnout. Cureus. 2018;10(7):e3076.
2. Miles SH. Hippocrates and informed consent. Lancet. 2009;374:1322–3.
3. Antoniou SA, Antoniou GA, Granderath FA, et al. Reflections of the Hippocratic oath in modern medicine. World J Surg. 2010;34(12):3075–9.
4. Jotterand F. The Hippocratic Oath and contemporary medicine: dialectic between past ideals and present reality? J Med Philos. 2005;30(1):107–28.
5. Sessanna L. Incorporating Florence Nightingale's theory of nursing into teaching a group of preadolescent children about the negative peer pressure. J Pediatr Nurs. 2004;19(3):225–31.
6. Beauchamp T, Childress J. Principles of biomedical ethics. 6th ed. New York: Oxford University Press; 2008.
7. Kuczmarski M, Adams E, Cotugna N, et al. Health literacy and education predict nutrient quality of diet of socioeconomically diverse, urban adults. J Epidemiol Prev Med. 2016;2(1):13000115.
8. Hoover DS, Vidrine JI, Shete S, et al. Health literacy, smoking, and health indicators in African American adults. J Health Commun. 2015;20(Suppl 2):24–33.
9. Baker DW, Parker RM, Williams MV, et al. The relationship of patient reading ability to self-reported health and use of health services. Am J Public Health. 1997;87(6):1027–30.

10. Bennett IM, Chen J, Soroui JS, White S. The contribution of health literacy to disparities in self-rated health status and preventive health behaviors in older adults. Ann Fam Med. 2009;7(3):204–11.
11. Berkman ND, Sheridan SL, Donahue KE, et al. Low health literacy and health outcomes: an updated systematic review. Ann Intern Med. 2011;155(2):97–107.
12. Berkman ND, Sheridan SL, Donahue KE, et al. Health literacy interventions and outcomes: an updated systematic review. Rockville: Agency for Healthcare Research and Quality; 2011.
13. Stewart DW, Vidrine JI, Shete S, et al. Health literacy, smoking, and health indicators in African American adults. J Health Commun. 2015;20(0 2):24–33.
14. Ogedegbe G, Harrison M, Robbins L, et al. Barriers and facilitators of medication adherence in hypertensive African Americans: a qualitative study. Ethn Dis. 2004;14(1):3–12.
15. Wilson RP, Freeman A, Kazda MJ, et al. Lay beliefs about high blood pressure in a low- to middle-income urban African-American community: an opportunity for improving hypertension control. Am J Med. 2002;112(1):26–30.
16. Dutta M, Sastry S, Dillard S, et al. Narratives of stress in health meanings of African Americans in Lake County, Indiana. Health Commun. 2017;32(10):1241–51.
17. Dubbin L, McLemore M, Shim JK. Illness narratives of African Americans living with coronary heart disease: a critical interactionist analysis. Qual Health Res. 2017;27(4):497–508.
18. Atreja A, Bellam N, Levy SR. Strategies to enhance patient adherence: making it simple. MedGenMed. 2005;7(1):4.
19. Rampersaud GC, Pereira MA, Girard BL, et al. Breakfast habits, nutritional status, body weight, and academic performance in children and adolescents. J Am Diet Assoc. 2005;105(5):743–60.
20. Fai EK, Anderson C, Ferreros V. Role of attitudes and intentions in predicting adherence to oral diabetes medications. Endocr Connect. 2017;6(2):63–70.
21. Rimando PM. Perceived barriers to and facilitators of hypertension management among underserved African American older adults. Ethn Dis. 2015;25(3):329.
22. Hardy ST, Loehr LR, Butler KR, et al. Reducing the blood pressure–related burden of cardiovascular disease: impact of achievable improvements in blood pressure prevention and control. J Am Heart Assoc. 2015;4(10):e002276.
23. Zhao W, Katzmarzyk PT, Horswell R, et al. HbA1c and coronary heart disease risk among diabetic patients. Diabetes Care. 2013;37(2):428–35.
24. Zhao W, Katzmarzyk PT, Horswell R, et al. HbA1c and lower-extremity amputation risk in low-income patients with diabetes. Diabetes Care. 2013;36(11):3591–8.
25. Woolf SH, Johnson RE, Fryer GE, et al. The health impact of resolving racial disparities: an analysis of US mortality data. Am J Public Health. 2004;94:2078–81.
26. Health Status & Life Expectancy. Black demographics. http://blackdemographics.com/health-2/health/. Accessed 25 May 2019.
27. African American Health. Centers for Disease Control and Prevention. 2017. https://www.cdc.gov/vitalsigns/aahealth/index.html. Accessed 25 may 2019.

Index

© Springer Nature Switzerland AG 2020   215
G. L. Hall, *Patient-Centered Clinical Care for African Americans*,
https://doi.org/10.1007/978-3-030-26418-5